Pilates and
Conditioning
for Athletes

An Integrated Approach
to Performance and Recovery

Amy Lademann
Rick Lademann

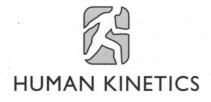

HUMAN KINETICS

Library of Congress Cataloging-in-Publication Data

Names: Lademann, Amy, 1972- author. | Lademann, Rick, 1974- author.
Title: Pilates and conditioning for athletes : an integrated approach to
    performance and recovery / Amy Lademann and Rick Lademann.
Description: Champaign, IL : Human Kinetics, [2019]
Identifiers: LCCN 2018031207 (print) | LCCN 2018036361 (ebook) | ISBN
    9781492557678 (ebook) | ISBN 9781492557661 (print)
Subjects: LCSH: Pilates method. | Athletes--Training of.
Classification: LCC RA781.4 (ebook) | LCC RA781.4 .L33 2019 (print) | DDC
    613.7/192--dc23
LC record available at https://lccn.loc.gov/2018031207

ISBN: 978-1-4925-5766-1 (print)

This publication is written and published to provide accurate and authoritative information relevant to the subject matter presented. It is published and sold with the understanding that the author and publisher are not engaged in rendering legal, medical, or other professional services by reason of their authorship or publication of this work. If medical or other expert assistance is required, the services of a competent professional person should be sought.

The web addresses cited in this text were current as of October 2018 unless otherwise noted.

Senior Acquisitions Editor: Michelle Maloney; **Developmental Editor:** Anne Hall; **Managing Editors:** Miranda K. Baur and Ann C. Gindes; **Copyeditor:** Annette Pierce; **Permissions Manager:** Martha Gullo; **Graphic Designer:** Julie L. Denzer; **Cover Designer:** Keri Evans; **Cover Design Associate:** Susan Rothermel Allen; **Photograph (cover):** Shutterstock/Ostill; **Photographs (interior):** Gregg Henness/ © Human Kinetics; **Photo Asset Manager:** Laura Fitch; **Photo Production Coordinator:** Amy M. Rose; **Photo Production Manager:** Jason Allen; **Senior Art Manager:** Kelly Hendren; **Illustrations:** © Human Kinetics; **Printer:** Versa Press

We thank Beyond Motion in Naples, Florida, for assistance in providing the location for the photo shoot for this book.

Human Kinetics books are available at special discounts for bulk purchase. Special editions or book excerpts can also be created to specification. For details, contact the Special Sales Manager at Human Kinetics.

Printed in the United States of America   10 9 8 7 6 5 4 3 2 1

The paper in this book is certified under a sustainable forestry program.

Human Kinetics
P.O. Box 5076
Champaign, IL 61825-5076
Website: www.HumanKinetics.com

In the United States, email info@hkusa.com or call 800-747-4457.
In Canada, email info@hkcanada.com.
In the United Kingdom/Europe, email hk@hkeurope.com.

For information about Human Kinetics' coverage in other areas of the world,
please visit our website: **www.HumanKinetics.com**

E7146

Pilates and Conditioning for Athletes

CONTENTS

Acknowledgments   v

Introduction   vii

PART I   PILATES CONDITIONING FOR YOUR BODY

1 **Functional Philosophy**   3

Pillars of performance frame the way to think about your training.

2 **Goal Setting, Primary Assessment, and Visualization**   17

Map out a plan for your ideal conditioning program.

3 **Daily Movements That Enhance Performance**   31

Learn how to fine-tune your movements for optimal performance.

4 **Movement Prep: Dynamic Warm-up**   73

Great workouts are built upon solid warm-up routines.

PART II   CONDITIONING EXERCISES

5 **Pilates Exercises**   97

Pilates exercises build the endurance and strength needed in all sports and every athletic discipline.

6 **Training With Medicine Balls and Resistance Bands**   155

Versatility is the hallmark of these overlooked fitness tools.

7 **Fundamental Strength Exercises**   195

Use barbells and dumbbells to push yourself to new levels.

PART III   THE WORKOUTS

8 Foundational Workouts 217

Structurally sound conditioning programs start with strong foundational workouts.

9 Intermediate, Advanced, and Sport-Specific Workouts 231

Progress your training based on your goals, sport, and level of conditioning.

Glossary   249

About the Authors   251

Earn Continuing Education Credits/Units   254

ACKNOWLEDGMENTS

This book is possible because of the amazing mentors and teachers we have had along the way. Without your ongoing encouragement and support we would not be where we are today.

Rick

Thank you, Al Vermeil, for taking me under your wing and teaching me a craft that I love. I am forever grateful. Thank you, Tim Adams, for always being a great friend and mentor in this field we love. Last, and definitely not least, thank you, Mom and Dad. You supported me from the beginning, always encouraging me throughout my journey while I was traveling around the country learning from the best of the best. Without you two none of this is possible.

Amy

I'd like to thank my family and friends for always encouraging me to do and be more. Thank you, Carmen Marshall, for reminding me anything and everything is possible. To all of our clients throughout the years, it's because of you that we strive to be the very best at what we do. And to Rick, you are always my inspiration. You have an amazing gift and to watch you coach, whether you're on the field or in the weight-room, is amazing. You have changed the lives of thousands of people and have inspired another generation of strength coaches. I love you!

Thank you to our Beyond Motion family for helping us with this project and constantly encouraging us when we were too tired to write another sentence. And to Heather for always checking in to make sure we had time to write. Wibs, Jamie, Kelly, Dom, and Carl, thank you for being such great models, you made it all so easy.

INTRODUCTION

*P*ilates and Conditioning for Athletes was written for you, the serious or elite athlete, or a coach working with high-level athletes. You will gain valuable insights and tips for training and recovery that will improve your level of play. We will provide you with pregame and postgame exercises to help you create a more functional system so that you will be able to better adapt to the demands placed on your body and perform at a higher level. As you read and use the assessment tests and training programs, you will follow programs similar to those that we use with the elite and professional athletes that train at our facility. Regardless of whether you are a 50-year-old triathlete, college athlete, professional athlete, or even a weekend warrior, this book has something for everyone.

We encourage you to follow the program completely, starting with your personal assessment tests. Once you have gone through each chapter, you will be able to select the individual workout at the end of the book based on your assessment, current needs, and goals. This is more than a book that you will read once and put on a shelf; *Pilates and Conditioning for Athletes* should be used as your training partner and coach. You will use this book whether you're working out at home, the gym, or on the road. As your results improve, refer back to the programs for inspiration and new workouts. You will be able to challenge yourself with a new workout every few months based on your performance level and needs at that time. Remember to log your progress and set your goals. Successful athletes never leave training to chance. They don't wander through their workout wondering, "What should I do next?" Every workout is planned. Every exercise is done for a specific reason, and each movement and program builds on the next.

This book is a culmination of more than two decades of inspiring work, research, and studying the training of professional and high-level athletes. Throughout the process we have learned that although each body is unique, every athlete requires the same fundamental strengths to perform at their highest level. The best athletes are strong, fast, reactive, and cognitively aware. To prepare you for competition, we have designed complete and balanced programs that tap into each of the key factors you need for success.

How did we go about doing this? Our philosophy is founded on a science-based approach, literally working with your body from the ground up, helping you to develop a more productive system both neurologically and in the musculature. This multidimensional training system, known as the seven pillars, will help you become a stronger, faster, healthier, and better-equipped athlete.

You will learn the benefits and basic techniques for the following:

- Breathing exercises for increased lung capacity, stress reduction, and breath control
- Stretching routines to open and lengthen your hips, hamstrings, and back
- Joint articulation to improve your range of motion and balance
- Ways to activate and strengthen your glutes
- A dynamic warm-up series to begin each session
- Myofascial release work to prepare your body for each program
- Pilates to strengthen your core, improve your posture, develop uniform strength, and increase flexibility
- Resistance training for strength and power exercises
- Medicine ball training for working in diagonal and transverse planes

Movement and Your Body

The fitness and conditioning community has seen lots of fads. One minute something is hot and considered to be "the best training method ever," and the next minute people are condemning the same program they once loved. There is a tendency to try to make things fancy and complicated, when in reality, all we need to do is return to the foundation of what makes an athlete faster and stronger. Every athlete has a weakness, and it is up to us as coaches to isolate those weaknesses and turn those areas into a strength.

Having trained athletes for about two decades, we have heard the same comments and questions time and again:

- "How do I know which exercises are best for me right now?"
- "My coach has been giving me the same workout for a long time. How do I know it's time to change?"
- "My body doesn't bounce back as quickly after workouts; what can I do?"
- "I stretch and I'm still so tight. What can I do?"
- "I'm injured . . . again. How do I prevent future injuries?"
- "What should I be doing in the off-season?"
- "I have heard that Pilates is a great workout, but how do I do it and when should I incorporate it?"

We are here to answer your questions. But first we need to explain what you will not see in this book. This book will not offer you a quick fix. It will not provide you with workout programs that are complicated and extreme. It will not push you past your breaking point and then criticize you for not pushing yourself hard enough.

What this book will do is coach you, guide you, and offer you opportunities to improve your athletic performance.

Debunk the Myths

This is the first book of its kind—one that not only dispels training myths and identifies inconsistencies in the world of athletic conditioning but also teaches you how to challenge your body in an entirely new way. Our method of overall conditioning for athletes is a multifaceted, tiered approach and works to help you create a strong, flexible base so that you can begin building on that foundation.

So what exactly will we teach you throughout this book? Well, the training for every athlete, no matter their sport or age, needs to use the same key components in order to be successful. These are our seven pillars of training: strength, flexibility, mobility, stability, power, speed, and agility.

Think about it. If you want to improve your speed, what factors do you need to address? Do you have a good strength base? Are you flexible? How is your mobility? How stable are you? Do you have good breath control and lung capacity? Without addressing these key factors, your ability to become faster is limited. Weak, inflexible athletes are not efficient movers. Our goal is to make sure your movement is efficient and effective, helping you reach your full athletic potential.

At our facility, an athlete's initial evaluation is the key to creating the ideal blueprint for his or her personalized training program. Once an evaluation is completed, we have a baseline to work from in order to create the initial training programs.

Our evaluation process places each athlete in a variety of situations that test their movement patterns, range of motion, strength base, flexibility, and core strength. At the end of the evaluation, we discuss the identified deficiencies and, more importantly, explain how we will address these factors one by one. Again, our goal is to turn these weaknesses into strengths, to keep our athletes on the field or court and off the bench.

Knowing that not everyone has the ability to train at our facility, we want to provide you with a way to become your own coach. We want to make sure you have the correct information and a simple format to use so that you are prepared to begin this phase of your training.

So where do you begin? How do you know which exercises are best suited for you to start with? This book provides step-by-step instructions for assessing your body so you can choose the best program to start with from the programs outlined at the back of the book. And then you'll reassess your body and program after 90 days. We will take the confusion out of conditioning and provide you with your own KISS (keep it super simple) method. You will learn our methodology of pre- and posttraining mechanics, Pilates, and overall conditioning so that no matter where you are, your program is available to you at all times. This is more than a what-to-do book.

This book provides you with a how-to-do-it plan. Within these pages you will find the answers your body has been asking for.

Once you take your initial assessment and read through the chapters, you will be able to determine which programs will best assist you right from the beginning. You will also be able to select the individual exercises that will help you reach your goals as well. We suggest following the same program for about 30 days, then retesting yourself using the same protocols as you did initially to check your progress. As you notice differences in your strength and performance, it might be time to add onto or change to another program.

PART I | PILATES CONDITIONING FOR YOUR BODY

1 | **Functional Philosophy**

Each of us performs hundreds of movements every day that serve a specific function or purpose. While we may use our entire body for some of those movements, such as getting out of bed in the morning or walking from one place to another, other movements require less body involvement: brushing our teeth, answering the phone, using our hands and arms to get food to our mouths. Most of the time, we don't have to think much about how we move. Our body functions according to patterns it has learned, and until we have an injury or limitation, that movement serves us well.

The term functional training, or functional fitness, refers to exercises or conditioning done to make our everyday movements more efficient and less likely to cause injury. It turns out that some of those repetitive actions we take, without thinking, might not be the most effective way to move and may cause or contribute to overuse injuries, strains, and more serious problems that, if not resolved, may lead to long-term muscular, joint, tissue, and nerve problems.

What does this mean for you as an athlete? Using a functional approach in your training can help you prevent those functional issues before they start, or address them so you can move the way you want. You may not have problems performing daily tasks such as getting out of bed or walking up the stairs, but is your body moving at its full potential? Are you at the top of your game in your chosen sport? Does your training program provide you with enough tools and knowledge to assist you in becoming a faster, stronger, more flexible, better-equipped athlete? If not, then this book is for you.

How Is Beyond Motion's Training Approach Different?

The Beyond Motion training philosophy looks at the body as one whole, functioning unit, addressing the weaknesses and strengthening the strengths. Everyone has their own genetic disposition; therefore, we truly are not all created equal. To help athletes reach their true potential, we designed our system of the seven pillars. As you become familiar with our system, you will not only learn how to address your own weaknesses, but you will also become more intuitive about your body, enabling you to become the athlete you envision.

Seven Pillars of Training

When we designed our facility and training programs, we were able to mesh our backgrounds to blend Pilates and athlete performance in a unique way. From so many years of working with professional, recreational, and student-athletes, we knew the areas athletes should focus on in order for their bodies to completely engage, and we based our training philosophy on developing those areas. Regardless of whether someone is a weekend athlete, an Ironman, or a professional baseball player, elite athletes share the same qualities.

All athletes possess some level of strength, flexibility, mobility, stability, power, speed, and agility, and great athletes possess them at high levels. It is a coach's job to determine which areas may be deficient and develop a program to improve them. For optimal performance, the components should be trained sequentially, starting with strength and ending with agility. As Michael Jordan once said, "My attitude is that if you push me towards something that you think is a weakness, then I will turn that perceived weakness into a strength." This quote inspired the formation of our concept of the seven pillars. If coaches address all seven pillars correctly, they will put athletes on the field who are ready to perform at their fullest genetic potential. The coach's job is to prepare the athlete. Taking a one-dimensional training approach is not coaching. Being knowledgeable enough to be adaptive and to see weaknesses and then having the tools to strengthen those weaknesses is the goal. So we'll start by going into more depth on the seven pillars concept.

Strength

Strength is the key that starts the car. The number one component an athlete needs is strength. Without strength, an athlete will fall short every time. There are two types of strength: relative strength and absolute strength. Relative strength is used during activities like walking and jogging. Absolute strength is built by external stimuli such as weightlifting. It's important that athletes understand the difference because often it is up to them and their team's strength coach to maintain their absolute strength. Unless an athlete is injured, relative strength will always be maintained because it occurs naturally without training. Absolute strength is the precursor to power. When a drop in absolute strength occurs, it is immediately noticeable on the field or court. Movement patterns break down and so does the athlete.

How do you measure strength? That's the key question when evaluating and developing athletes. Simple tests such as the one repetition maximum (1RM) squat test can be effective and valuable. The goal weight for a male athlete's 1RM squat is close to two times his body weight. A male athlete who weighs 180 pounds (82 kg) should squat about 350 pounds (159 kg). The goal for women is 1.5 times their body weight, so a 135-pound (61 kg) woman should squat 200 pounds (91 kg) or more. These are aggressive numbers, but to compete at full potential, an athlete needs to meet these benchmarks. It is not unusual for the athlete with the highest 1RM squat and clean to also be the best athlete on the field or court. When Beyond Motion athlete Chris Sale, who pitches for the Boston Red Sox, trains during the off-season, he focuses on the strength pillar because it is his biggest need for both conditioning and Pilates. After five off-seasons of training, he is achieving this goal, and he is therefore more consistent in his movement patterns off the mound.

Flexibility

This is a tough one. Most people love to train but hate to stretch. Athletes need supple tissue; think tenderloin, not sirloin. Elastic tissue creates fluid

Mobility Created

Larry Walker, Colorado Rockies National League MVP, provides a great example of how improvements in flexibility can improve performance. In the early 2000s, Larry experienced multiple injuries. Although he was an extremely well-rounded athlete, he was tight through the hips and hamstrings. It was not clear whether this was caused by previous injuries, but it was clear that flexibility had to be the number one priority. Pilates wasn't used extensively with athletes at that time, but proprioceptive neuromuscular facilitation (PNF) stretching methods provided a solution to Larry's flexibility needs. As an example, when Larry completed a set of Romanian deadlifts, he followed them with antagonistic quadriceps stretches on a table with a trainer. This process trained the muscles on the back of his body, or posterior chain, while making sure he developed the full range of motion in his hip flexors, where he experienced a lot of inhibition. Using this technique with his hamstring and hips created our next pillar, mobility.

movement and, most importantly, limits injuries. Flexibility creates fluidity, and fluidity is responsible for the beauty in sports. Everyone is flexible to some extent. Athletes at the low end of the scale are generally more injury **prone.** If you watch closely, you'll see that their movements are mechanical, and their movement patterns on the field or court lack of fluidity.

Mobility

What is mobility? Everyone talks about it, but what does mobility contribute on the field of play? Let's start with this: Flexibility involves the length of a muscle, while mobility affects how a joint moves through a range of motion. Let's go back to Larry Walker. The lack of flexibility in his hips affected his mobility. Flexibility and mobility are symbiotic. Conversely, an athlete can be so flexible that mobility becomes an issue because of lack of strength.

Coaching Tip

During our initial evaluation with Major League pitcher Bronson Arroyo, it was clear that he had been a workhorse on the mound for many years. He was what in baseball is called an inning eater: someone who can go deep in the game and save their bullpen's arms. As a seasoned pitcher constantly working at his maximum capacity, the excessive volume of pitching and training became an issue. His muscle tissue was tense and not as supple as we like to see. It may surprise you, but we are referring to his hips and not his arm. When we conducted an external rotation test on both hips, we discovered that Bronson had a very hard end point, meaning that the tissue locked up and proper movement was inhibited, which caused compensation in other areas of the body. Ideally, you want to feel some give in the last few degrees of abduction (moving away from the body), and in Bronson's case, his tissue wasn't able to release. During the evaluation it was also clear that Bronson had an abundance of absolute strength. He had been lifting his entire athletic life and he enjoyed having a heavy weight on his back. He had responded well to this form of training throughout his career and had prospered because of it.

The next step was explaining to Bronson that being in the weight room would not be his first priority during that off-season. It was apparent that addressing his flexibility and tissue issues through massage and active release therapy (ART) should be the first step in his program. Once he developed a greater range of movement, he was able to return to the style of lifting he was accustomed to.

As performance coaches, it's up to us to prioritize off-season needs even when the athletes won't be happy about it. Sometimes it takes a paradigm shift for athletes to realize that their priorities will change as they continue to mature and grow in their sport. Mobility was our first priority, and we needed to make sure Bronson understood that this was a change he needed to make. After explaining the pillars to Bronson, he grasped the importance of it instantly. He's a cognitive athlete, and understanding the necessity allowed him to put himself in the best frame of mind to work toward his goals.

Therefore we go back to our first and most important pillar: strength. Now you're seeing how these three tie together. It takes a coach's eye to gauge an athlete's level of strength, flexibility, and mobility and understand how they affect each other and performance. The more you work with athletes, the easier it will become to accurately evaluate these components.

Stability

When we discuss stability in relation to an athlete, we're not necessarily referring to a bigger, heavier athlete being more stable because they have greater mass. We are referring to how stable an athlete is in their movement patterns. Are they able to get into and hold a particular position or movement because their muscles are working together correctly, or is their body going into compensation mode due to weakness, thereby creating instability? Sometimes we see instability in athletes with poor muscle tissue and extra tightness. Other times instability is coming from injury and compensations. As coaches, it is our job to determine where the instability is coming from and address it accordingly.

Your glutes drive your knees, meaning the power that comes from your glutes helps stabilize your knee joints. If you are unable to stabilize the front of the knee during a lunge, it is a clear indication that your glutes are not firing, and this weakness is causing instability at the knee and hip. Let's dig into this a bit. The glutes drive the knees, the knees drive the ankles, and the ankles drive the feet. Can you see the chain of events occurring now? If one of those areas lacks strength and stability, you're experiencing something we refer to at Beyond Motion as *leakage*. Leakage, in this case, means that you're leaking through one of the joints during the movement and lacking the control required for that position. Essentially, you're wasting energy. By developing greater stability in all of those joints, you will notice an improvement in overall movement patterns and be able to execute a clean, smooth movement.

Defying Logic

Winston Justice, a former NFL lineman, was referred to us after knee arthroscopy. Our first priority was to get his glutes and posterior chain to fire in order to take pressure off the knees and stabilize them so he could get a few more years out of the joint. After working with him, he was able to play for another three years before retirement, so we were successful. Winston is a great example of someone who was able to play simply because his lower half was so strong that he defied logic. His pillar of strength created the stability he had no business having. That strength allowed Winston to experience minimal leakage so that his power output was consistently high.

Power

Power is the ability to create force. You can't create force without having a great strength base. An athlete who is 5' 9" and can dunk a basketball has already established a solid foundation of strength that she is able to use when jumping vertically. This means that the athlete understands how to create power. Power results from developing the previous pillars and engaging flexibility, mobility, and strength all at once.

Speed

Speed is one of the most sought after traits in an athlete. Speed is the ability to cover distance in a particular amount of time. It is a learned skill that many athletes spend little time perfecting. Speed comes from within, meaning that even if an athlete is coached all day long on the track, and the athlete may understand the process of gaining speed, there is also a feel component required by the athlete to perfect this skill. It's the reps you take when no one is watching that really count. It's the reps that feel rhythmic and smooth that carry over. You can't increase speed by training this skill at anything under 99 percent. Speed work is the most draining of all training forms on your nervous system, and we are always looking for quality not quantity. Therefore it must be strategically phased into an athlete's program. When training someone to increase their speed, there are several components from the seven pillars that come into play including strength, agility, mobility, and flexibility. To become fast, athletes must develop a strength

---

Rick's Tips

I had the great opportunity to spend two years working under the direction of weightlifting coach Dragomir Cioroslan at the Olympic Training Center in Colorado Springs. Cioroslan was a 1984 Olympic bronze medalist, representing Romania. During this time I was able to watch and coach some of the most powerful athletes in the United States. It was in that old plane hangar at the OTC coaching Olympic lifting when I said to myself, "This is how you create power." So this pillar holds a lot of special memories for me.

Olympic lifting is included in all of our athletes' programs and is one of the key elements of our programming. Athletes drive through the ground in order to create force. The perfect mechanism to prepare an athlete for this is performing Olympic lifts, specifically a clean or a snatch. Both movements require a high power output and have a strong eccentric phase, meaning absorbing and stabilizing the bar during the catch. To perform the lifts correctly, athletes must master the propulsion aspect of the lift as well as the absorption of the negative component. A negative component is learning how to decelerate, whether it be your speed or a barbell.

---

base first. As they're building their base, they or their coach should be able to identify which of the seven pillars need to be addressed in order for them to develop greater speed.

Agility

Have you had the opportunity to watch tennis professional Roger Federer play in person? If you haven't and you're in the performance field, it's a must. His movement is effortless, and he embodies the agility pillar. Agility can be described as the ability to move quickly and easily. So here's the big question: Can you train agility? Some coaches say you either have it or you don't. We believe everyone has their own predisposition for it, but you can train it. Agility has a neurological component that should be addressed starting at an early age. It is also important in an athlete's off-season training program. It may take athletes many weeks or months to see improvement in their speed and agility. And agility, much like power, has many influences. You cannot be agile without flexibility, strength, mobility, and power. When all components mesh, you get a pure, beautiful movement. Coaches may work with agile athletes, but is their agility the best it can be? Remember, a coach's job is to bring out the best in their athletes. Nothing else will be tolerated.

With the seven pillars in place, coaches have a comprehensive system that they can refer to when evaluating an athlete's deficiencies and strengths and determining what the athlete needs. They don't need to re-create the wheel. A great example of finding strengths and weaknesses comes from Al Vermeil, strength coach for the Chicago Bulls. When he was asked whether he trained players by incorporating a variety of plyometrics into their programs, his answer often surprised people. The fact of the matter was, very little plyometric work was added to their program. He saw no need to repeat a pattern the players had been performing all day as they played basketball. What they did not spend all day doing was strength training and Olympic lifting. Which pillars were missing? Strength and power. By focusing their training on these components, he developed even stronger, more explosive athletes on the court.

To develop our seven pillars, we use a modality that combines them, something that will help you become an even more in-tune athlete. It is one of our secret weapons, and it is Pilates.

What Is Pilates?

Pilates, originally called Contrology, was created by Joseph Pilates. In his 1945 book, *Return to Life Through Contrology*, he presents his method as "the art of controlled movements, which should look and feel like a workout (not a therapy) when properly manifested." When practiced with consistency,

Pilates will improve your flexibility, build greater strength, and will help you to develop balance, control, and endurance within your entire body. The core, consisting of the muscles of the abdomen, low back, and hips, is often referred to as your powerhouse. Think of it as the key to your stability. We can modify Pilates exercises from beginner to advanced, as well as develop programs based on your goals and limitations. The intensity of your Pilates workout will increase over time as your body adapts.

Principles of Pilates

Although there is no mention of Joseph Pilates listing an order of principles for Contrology, over the years instructors have keyed in on six focal points used within each exercise, regardless of whether the exercise is performed on the floor or any of the pieces of Pilates equipment.

We'll go into more detail about how to incorporate these principles directly into your athletic training in chapter 5.

Six Pilates Principles

1. Breathing—This releases stress from your body, creates a deeper connection to your core, and releases stiffness within your spine.
2. Centering—By physically bringing your focus to the center of your body, also known as your powerhouse, you feel the connection between the front and back of the body, and from your ribs to your pubic bone.
3. Concentration—By staying present in what you are doing at that moment you can focus on each exercise and its purpose.
4. Coordination—Coordinating your brain and body, and your breath and your movement, increases your brain's control of your body's movement and dynamic function.
5. Flow—Each Pilates movement should be smooth and fluid. The exercises should flow from one movement to the next without the feeling of stopping and starting each exercise.
6. Precision (otherwise known as control)—Work with flow, not momentum. Control, rather than intensity or repetition, is key to performing the exercises correctly. Perform all of your movements with precision to gain the maximum benefits.

Pilates in Real Life

Every day, professional and recreational athletes enter our facility looking for something more: a competitive edge, more knowledge, or something to help them feel and perform better. To help them achieve their goals, after initial evaluation, we include Pilates in the training programs we implement.

The Story of Joseph Hubertus Pilates

Joseph Pilates was born December 9, 1883 in Mönchengladbach (near Düsseldorf), Germany. His Greek father was a prize-winning gymnast and his German mother was said to be a naturopath.

As a child, Joseph had asthma and contracted rickets and rheumatic fever. He was determined to overcome his ailments, and, at a young age, researched ways to become bigger, stronger, and healthier. He educated himself in anatomy, bodybuilding, wrestling, yoga, gymnastics, and martial arts. Over time, he developed an almost Adonis-like body. His physique was so developed that at the age of 14, he posed for anatomy charts.

Joseph was enamored by the classical Greek ideals of a man, someone who was balanced equally in body, mind, and spirit. He was convinced that the modern lifestyle, bad posture, and inefficient breathing were the root of poor health. To combat these problems, he designed a series of exercises that incorporated his vast knowledge of the human body to correct muscular imbalances and improve posture, coordination, balance, strength, and flexibility as well as to increase breathing capacity and organ function.

In 1914, after World War I broke out, he was interned along with other German nationals in a camp for enemy aliens in Lancaster, England. It was at this time that he began devising a system of original exercises and called this regimen Contrology, meaning the complete coordination of the body, mind, and spirit. During this time, Joseph refined his ideas and trained others to perform his exercises. He rigged springs to hospital beds, which allowed bedridden patients to exercise using the resistance to create stability or mobility depending on the case. Following his release at the war's end in 1918, Joseph returned to Germany and continued to refine his fitness methods. Word of his success grew and he was hired by the city of Hamburg to train their policemen.

In 1926, Joseph immigrated to the United States. He met his future wife, Clara, on the boat to New York City. Together they opened the first Contrology studio in Manhattan, in the same building as several dance studios. Joseph's studio became the place dancers went to rehabilitate their injuries and train. They were sent to him to be "fixed."

Joseph was both inventive and resourceful and spent the rest of his life perfecting the art of Contrology, now known as Pilates. He designed and crafted many pieces of equipment that we still use today in Pilates studios and physical therapy facilities around the world. Spring tension is used for resistance or assistance, straps hold feet or hands, supports and pads hold the back, neck, and shoulders in correct alignment. Pilates equipment is a great complement to the Pilates mat work, which is considered more difficult for some people than Pilates exercises on the equipment. During Pilates mat work you rely on your body's own strength and flexibility to perform each move, and the springs on the Pilates equipment provide both the assistance and resistance needed for each of the Pilates exercises.

Joseph died in 1967 of advanced emphysema from smoking cigars for too many years. Clara continued to teach and run the studio until she passed away in 1977. The exercises they originally designed are still used as models for the work we do today. Each exercise has a stability piece and a mobility piece, and the fluidity of each movement increases endurance, breath control, strength, and flexibility. All key pieces enhance the quality of movement for athletes and nonathletes alike. Pilates is one of the only comprehensive exercise programs in which you work and stretch simultaneously instead of working out first and stretching after.

Today, millions of people use Pilates as not only a form of therapy, but also as a main component of their training program. What a great testament to Joseph Pilates. He really was someone who was ahead of his time.

Our athletes often tell us that after their initial Pilates session they are amazed at how much easier all of their other training throughout the week feels. They feel longer and more open, move with greater body awareness, and feel an increased sense of focus and ease. Just like in any program or sport, understanding the fundamentals is exceptionally important.

These are the first five things we teach all new students:

1. Pilates is Pilates. Any other exercise form combined with Pilates is no longer Pilates. The Pilates mat work is the foundation for all of the other exercises performed on all pieces of Pilates equipment. Because you rely on your own body's strength and flexibility, it may also be the most challenging group of exercises to learn and perform well. Because the spring tension on the Pilates equipment can be used to add resistance and increase assistance, many exercises may seem easier to learn and perfect on the equipment than on the floor.

2. As you learn the exercises and increase your knowledge, your movements will become more fluid and can be done with greater precision. We use flow, not momentum, and precision, not rigidity. We do not operate in the world of reps and sets. Many Pilates exercises are repeated no more than eight times before you move onto the next exercise within your program.

3. Every Pilates exercise should have a work or strength component and a flexibility component.

4. A part of your body is always creating stability while you are working mobility at the other end.

5. Not every exercise can be performed by every person in the same way. Injuries, compensations, weaknesses, and tightness create areas of your body that don't work as well as others do. Modifications and the use of props to get your body into the correct form may be necessary.

Pilates Principles and the Seven Pillars

Pilates is a complete body-conditioning program that integrates your mind and body to improve precision in muscle control, strength, flexibility, and breath control. Joseph himself described his system of Contrology as "a method of physical and mental conditioning." The exercises within the Pilates repertoire help to activate lesser-used muscles and require full recruitment of your core (powerhouse). The movements work to develop more symmetrical muscle development, allowing you to work more efficiently and effectively.

Stability and Mobility

As mentioned earlier, each Pilates exercise incorporates a component of both stability and mobility. Integrating these components helps to create fluid movements that feel as if they glide from one exercise to another rather than a constant sensation of stopping one movement and then starting another. Think of Pilates as a way to create space and length within your body. It will open your joints, elongate your muscles, deepen your breath control, build your endurance, and connect your mind to your body. Your Pilates practice will help you to create an entirely new relationship with your body.

Flexibility

Pilates can correct body imbalances caused by injury or postural problems by aligning the body correctly and balancing the muscular and external forces affecting the joints, muscles, and skeleton. We use Pilates as an integral part of rehabilitation from overuse or misuse of the body, helping athletes reduce their chance of additional injuries postrecovery. We often find that many athletes' injuries are caused not only by weakness and compensation, but also by muscle tightness. By incorporating Pilates into their weekly program, they are able to increase their range of motion and enhance their overall flexibility.

Agility

Pilates will help to increase your spatial awareness and body control. These new patterns are fine-tuned through repetition and are directly transferable to the gym, field, court, course, or track.

Power

Pilates will help you increase your power output. Your body cannot generate power from a position of instability. Increased core stability is one of the key benefits of every Pilates program, enabling you to channel and maximize your power more efficiently and effectively. As your body develops greater strength and stability through your hips and core, you will be able to generate greater power and force. Many exercises mimic specific patterns along the kinetic chain that are used in movements on the field and court. The National Academy of Sports Medicine defines the kinetic chain as the relationship or connection between your nerves, muscles, and bones. The kinetic chain is broken into two categories, the open kinetic chain and the closed kinetic chain, and is used to help describe or classify exercises. For example, when you squat, your foot presses against the floor to raise and lower your body. This is a closed kinetic chain exercise. Using a leg curl machine, where the lower leg swings freely, is an example of an open kinetic chain exercise.

Strength and Speed

Pilates exercises such as the side-lying leg series place people in unilateral positions. By working through similar exercises, you discover how to balance your body's weaknesses and find greater symmetry and strength from your right to left side, and from the front to back of your body. Strength and flexibility have a direct correlation to speed. When athletes have a strong base and their muscles are "elastic" and flexible, they are more likely to increase their speed. Weak and tight muscles limit speed.

Benefits for Elite Athletes

Take a moment to think about how the bodies of most elite swimmers look. Typically, they look strong, their musculature appears thicker than that of other athletes, and their posture is more forward and their shoulders rounded. Now in comparison, picture a ballerina. Ballet dancers tend to appear taller than they are. Their posture is more elevated, and while they are strong and muscular, they appear long and lean. Obviously, the postures of the two are quite different, as are their musculature and training.

One of our athletes was a talented high school swimmer. She spent her life in the pool and gym. Practice began as early as 5:00 a.m., and most of the time she trained twice a day. She was driven, focused, and willing to do whatever her coaches asked of her. As you can imagine, while she was amazing in the pool, her body had been put through the wringer. Over the years we worked to balance her anterior and posterior sides, enhance core strength, improve her flexibility and posture, create greater flexibility in the lower half, and deepen her breath control. This work helped to increase her body awareness both in and out of the pool. The changes in her overall composition were amazing. Her flexibility, compared to when she began her Pilates program, was unbelievable. She gained a significant amount of flexibility in her mid- and upper-**thoracic spine** as well as her hamstrings. Her chest and shoulders became more open, and her range of motion throughout her shoulder girdle increased. She noticed a decrease in her overall recovery time and a significant improvement in her core strength, all of which helped her improve her race times. In 2017, she committed to swim for the Georgia Bulldogs, an NCAA Division 1 program, and hopes to continue to incorporate Pilates into her training program.

Benefits for Recreational Athletes

While Pilates offers clear and important advantages for elite athletes, the benefits are equally valuable for recreational athletes. In fact, we see more injuries and postural issues in recreational athletes than in pros.

Unless they are an elite or professional athlete, most people do not train or work out as part of their career. Most people have fairly sedentary jobs.

Many of our clients train or play their favorite sports for a few hours each week, followed up with many hours on the phone; at a computer; or traveling in a car, train, or plane. This is a recipe for tight muscles, poor posture, and body imbalances. Pilates is the perfect complement to any training program. Think of Pilates as the antidote for the rest of your life.

"By starting Pilates, my fitness level, core strength, and flexibility have greatly increased. This has helped my overall quality of life and with my hobbies of tennis, kayaking, and biking. Combining my Pilates sessions with my conditioning program has helped my overall leg strength, mobility, and recovery from knee surgery."

—Terry North, client and lifelong athlete

Relationship Between Pilates and Resistance Training

Pilates and resistance training have a symbiotic relationship. Lifting weights is actually a neurologically driven movement working against external forces on your body while maintaining internal stability. The patterns of what we do under tension are for a specific amount of time or a specific number of reps. Pilates is similar in the sense that it uses the stabilizing muscles in movement patterns using internal forces, but it demands fluidity. While these may sound similar, Pilates and resistance training have two different applications on our central nervous system. Weightlifting heightens the sympathetic nervous system, which is a response to stress on the body. Pilates heightens the parasympathetic nervous system, which slows the heart rate and relaxes the musculature within it. These two methods together create balance in your body that cannot be duplicated. Put them together in your training program and you will notice very quickly that your body moves with a greater sense of ease because you will be able to balance the two components of the central nervous system. Either component tends to be overtrained if you focus on just one or the other.

All wins happen because the players on a team are prepared. The coach created a game plan and each player knew their role and perfected their skills. What is your goal? Is it to become stronger? Do you need to improve your flexibility and mobility? Are you working to become faster? Are you recovering from an injury and need to improve your agility and stability? Whatever your goal, the next several chapters provide a road map to help you get there.

Next Steps

Knowing not everyone will be able to hop on a plane to Florida for a personal evaluation and to train at Beyond Motion, we want to teach you how to apply the seven pillars and Pilates principles so you can create your personal game plan. Allow us to coach you or your team so you will increase your wins. In the following chapters you will find a self-assessment that will allow you to evaluate yourself to see what your body needs now.

Remember, success only happens when a well-thought-out game plan is executed. So once you have read though each chapter to learn about the tools you need to reach your personal best, it is up to you to find the program at the end of the book that works best for you and to follow it.

2 | Goal Setting, Primary Assessment, and Visualization

Some young athletes spend their entire lives working toward huge goals. They know from the time they are very young that they want to be an Olympic athlete and are willing to do anything and everything it takes to reach their dream. Their goal setting is based on achieving their dream. They may be too young to know the details of what goal setting is, but they know they need to focus, work hard, and listen to their coaches and that there are many steps between where they are now and where they want to be. If they are talented and work hard enough they may end up training at the Olympic Training Center in Colorado Springs, Colorado.

At the Olympic Training Center (OTC), coaches are in charge of just one team instead of many. The coaches and athletes have the same goal: make the Olympic team and compete in the games. For these athletes to qualify for the team and be prepared, they needed to make the most of the four years leading up to the Olympic games. Athletes who do not have a reasonable chance to make the team are either asked to leave or they willingly drop out of the program. The athletes who are competitive enough to have a chance to make the team become the coaches' main focus. In the 1990s, I spent two years living and working at the OTC in Colorado Springs working with USA Weightlifting.

One might think the stiff competition in this atmosphere would be detrimental for the American Olympic weightlifting team, but it was just the opposite. It drove these athletes to compete and sacrifice like never before. It brought out the best in these young lifters, coaches, and the program. Today the United States has a much stronger hold on Olympic weightlifting success than it did years ago.

Why Goals?

The weightlifters at the OTC knew their goal. They worked hard to get to where they were, they knew how much time they had to prepare, and they knew what they needed to do once they reached the OTC. You aren't invited to the OTC to be a part of the Olympic weightlifting team unless you have impressive clean, jerk, and snatch totals. Each team member worked toward their goals to beat their personal best and make the team. And head Olympic weightlifting coach, Dragomir Cioroslan, was skilled at working with each athlete to help them set and reach their short-term goals. He had a knack for understanding what motivated each of his team members.

Dragomir set specific goals for each athlete, and the athletes knew what was expected of them. This is a great example of how high-end athletes set their goals. However, few people have the benefit of a coach in their ear twice a day. That's why it's important to know how to set your goals by creating microcycles. This means that every six weeks you set a short-term goal that is a step toward where you want to be long term. For any athlete in any sport, it is important to understand the long-term plan. Working in small blocks of six-week cycles helps keep you focused and engaged while you work toward your ultimate outcome.

Setting Goals

What do you want to achieve? What are your long- and short-term goals? Setting short-term parameters keeps you feeling engaged and accomplished as you progress. Motivation, focus, consistency, and confidence are essential when trying to reach any type of goal. You need a road map of what you want to accomplish in measureable terms and a plan so that you know what to do in order to get there. Setting goals and creating your road map are crucial parts of your training process.

> "If you don't know where you're going, you might not get there."
> —Yogi Berra

Goals will keep you both aware of your mission and focused on your outcome. When setting yours, or helping your athletes set theirs, make sure your goals are SMART: specific, measureable, attainable, relative, and time oriented.

Coaching Tip

If your job is to train athletes, you have to find ways to get them to understand that working toward their goal is a marathon and not a sprint. Short-term goals are essential to getting them to buy in to the program.

Let's use a vertical jump as an example. Explain to an athlete that the higher they jump, the more force they will be able to apply. Because a prerequisite of force is strength, as their vertical jump increases, it confirms that they not only are getting stronger, but becoming more powerful as well. As the athlete sees the results, they begin to recognize the importance of short-term goals. Clarifying this process for your athletes is key, and they will need to hear it time and time again. Remember: It takes many consistent reps to create a solid understanding of the process.

Specific

Your goals should be clear and easy to understand.

- What is the desired outcome?
- The short-term goals have to be clearly stated.
- You need to believe in these goals and be prepared to work to achieve them.

Measurable

How will you measure the short- and long-term progressions?

- Set test dates ahead of time that keep you accountable.
- Celebrate every small success; this will pump energy into your program.
- Numbers are essential for gauging your progress as an athlete. Coaches and general managers want to see them, too.

Attainable

All goals must present a challenge while being attainable.

- It's good to shoot for the stars, but don't be too extreme. Likewise, a goal that is too easy to meet will not motivate you. Only you know your limits.
- You'll find that many tiny steps in goal setting lead to success in reaching larger goals.

Relevant

Set goals that are important to where you are in your life right now. Setting a goal that someone else pressures you to attain will not be motivating.

- Examine your progress toward your goal so far. Is your goal still relevant to you?
- Does it excite you?
- Without passion we have nothing, so it's essential that athletes be excited and passionate enough that reaching their goal can become a reality.

Time Oriented

Include an end point. Knowing that you have a deadline will motivate you to get started.

- Because your training schedule will affect your outcome, begin far enough in advance to reach your goal, but not so far ahead that you lose focus.
- Know where your starting point is. For example, if you are trying to improve your finish time in a race, when was your last race? What was your time? How did you feel before and after the event? What are you hoping to accomplish with your new training program?

Types of Goals

You have confirmed what you want to accomplish. Now let's discuss the types of goals that are most helpful to athletes. We've all heard or created goals in terms of short-term, long-term, and lifetime, but have you thought about outcome goals, performance goals, and process goals?

Outcome Goals

These goals are determined by the specific results you want from an event or competition. It is what you're working toward. An outcome goal in a race

Coaching Tip

To help your athletes set realistic goals, you will need data. So your first day of training with a new team should be a test day. Record their weight, height, vertical leap, shuttle time, and 10-yard (9 m), 20-yard (18 m), and 40-yard (36 m) sprint times. The tests should be easily repeated under the same conditions. It takes a lot of effort to test, so you may be tempted to skip it. Our advice: Do it even if the set-up is extensive and time consuming. Testing every six weeks keeps coaches, managers, and athletes informed and pleased with progress.

might be stated as "I want to take 3 minutes off my finish time in my next 10K race, which is three months from now." Even developing the mindset of whether you are going to win or lose a race is establishing an outcome goal.

Performance Goals

What you are trying to achieve? It is important to measure and track in writing your starting point and how you are doing along the way. We tend to forget what we do not write down. It is easy to forget the path it took to reach the goal once the goal is achieved. Think of a performance goal as being one that you have the ability to control. You are in charge of your attitude, energy, work ethic and, in turn, your overall performance. Establishing your own clear, concise performance statements that keep you on track to reach your goals is important. Creating statements that reflect your short-term goals should be part of your performance goals versus outcome goals. Remember, your performance goals focus on your personal performance while outcome goals focus strictly on your outcome or result. The best way to measure your progress is by looking back at where you began and comparing it to where you are today. This is more helpful than comparing your success to someone else's.

Process Goals

These goals describe the steps you will take and the training you will complete to reach your performance and outcome goals. For example, your goal may be to lift weights for 45 minutes, five days a week for a month in order to gain 5 pounds (2.3 kg) of muscle mass in three months.

Process goals work well because instead of setting specific outcomes you want to achieve, you are creating the conditions in which you will work toward your long-term goals. Developing a process by which to attain your goals helps reduce the feeling that the big, long-term goals are almost unattainable. The specific steps are easier to manage along the way.

Assessing Your Goals

When setting your goals, remember to list the largest goal first. What are you working toward? Do you want to increase your endurance during postseason training, or do you want to take minutes off your upcoming marathon time? Next, think about the steps necessary to get where you want to go. How will you track your progress? How will you measure progress as you go? Last, how will you get to that place? Do you have someone to train with who specializes in the area you want to improve? What will you do every day to bring yourself one step closer to the goal you're working toward?

In most cases, once you know the outcome you're striving for and the performance requirements you need to get there, things move easily. Remember: The most important focus is the process.

Not only is knowing where you're going important, but it is also important to recognize (but not focus on) the obstacles that may come your way in your pursuit of your goals. Schedules change and injuries happen, but keeping a focus on your end goal allows you to be able to handle whatever comes your way and plan accordingly.

Keeping a written list of your goals helps you focus on what you want to achieve and remain realistic about how long it will take to get there. You may want to copy the Goal Checklist on page 23 so that you can reuse it every time you set a new goal for yourself.

Physical Assessment

Now that you have identified your goal, established realistic actions surrounding your goal, and can actually see yourself reaching your goal, it's time to evaluate your current physical status so you can plan your training accordingly.

You can use the form on page 27 to record your assessment results. Answer each question honestly and remember that today is day one. Everyone has a starting point, so be as accurate as possible. That will help you to create practical and realistic plans for reaching your goal. While we take regular assessments here at our facility, we suggest that people check in and reevaluate their status every 30 days. If they are following their program, they will be able to see and feel progress within 30 days.

Measurements

Weight is one assessment tool used whether you are looking to lose weight or gain weight or muscle. Measuring the circumference of various parts of your body is also important for providing an overall view of your starting point.

Measure circumference with a soft tape measure. Stand with your legs about hip-distance apart and weight evenly distributed on your right and left side. For the most accurate results, someone else should take your measurements.

Tips

- When measuring the chest, place the tape measure across the nipple line, centering it across the shoulder blades.
- When measuring the biceps, make sure the tape is at the center or widest portion of the upper arm above the elbow.
- Waist measurements should be taken slightly below the lowest rib and across the navel.
- Hips should be measured at their widest point, which typically falls at about the center of the glutes.

Goal Checklist

Today's date: _____

Long-term goal: _____

_____

Date to achieve long-term goal: _____

Why this goal is important to me:_____

_____

_____

Top three short-term goals to help me reach my long-term goal:

    1. _____

    2. _____

    3. _____

The time frame in which they will be achieved: _____

_____

My strengths (experiences, skills, and resources) that will help me reach my goals:

_____

_____

_____

My weaknesses (limitations, areas to improve, resources I don't have) I need to overcome to achieve my goals:

_____

_____

_____

Threats (time constraints, obstacles) that might hinder reaching my goals:

_____

_____

_____

Strengths I possess that could help reduce these identified threats:

_____

_____

_____

My reward for reaching my short-term and long-term goals:

_____

_____

_____

From A. Lademann and R. Lademann, *Pilates and Conditioning for Athletes: An Integrated Approach to Performance and Recovery* (Champaign, IL: Human Kinetics, 2019).

- Standing with legs apart, thighs should be measured at the fullest part.
- Calves should be measured at the widest point.

Body Fat

Measuring body fat is important. Skinfold measurements are taken using calipers on several areas of your body (see figure 2.1). It's best if someone else takes this reading because it can be challenging to get into the best position for an accurate reading when using calipers on yourself. Use the same calipers and, if possible, the same helper every time you measure your body fat. Just like every scale is different, each set of calipers is slightly different and may produce a different reading. Your goal is to record consistent measurements.

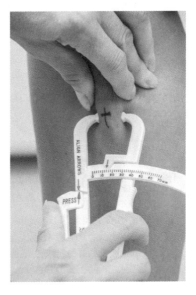

FIGURE 2.1   Skin calipers.

When performing a skinfold test, the idea is to pinch and pull. Attempt to separate the fat tissue from the surrounding tissue with a good pinch, and then pull it away from the body slightly.

Testing for Men

- Chest: Find the midpoint between your nipple and the crease of the armpit.
- **Abdominals**: Make a vertical fold 1 inch (2.5 cm) to the right of your navel.
- Thigh: Find the midpoint between the hip and the knee and use a vertical fold.

Testing for Women

- Triceps: Find the midpoint between the bony knob on top of your shoulder and the point of the elbow.
- Iliac crest: This site is below the lowest rib at the top ridge of the hipbone, called the iliac crest.
- Thigh: Measure at the midpoint between the hip and the knee.

Taking Skinfold Measurements

1. Pinch a skinfold with the thumb and index finger.
2. Place the measuring tips of the calipers at a right angle, pinch, and wait 2 seconds.
3. Note and record the reading.

4. Release the calipers.
5. Wait 1 to 2 seconds, and repeat two more times.
6. Add the three measurements and obtain the average by dividing the number by 3.
7. Repeat this process for each body area.

How to Read Skinfold Test Results

- In general for men, a score of 80 or lower is excellent and a score of 150 or higher is poor.
- A score for a woman of 90 or lower is excellent and a score of 150 or higher is poor.

Primary Assessments

In each of the following tests, give yourself a pass or fail. If you need to improve in an area so that you pass a test, you will find guidelines for how to improve in chapter 3.

Strength

Can you squat your body weight 10 times? If you can complete more than 10 repetitions, it's a strong pass. If this is not attainable, then you need to work on it. Remember: Your lower half is essential in every sport.

Speed

How fast can you run 40 yards (36 m)? If you score 5.2 seconds or less, you pass this test. Over 5.2 seconds could indicate a lack of power and strength and an area for improvement.

Power

If your vertical jump is 22 inches (56 cm) or higher, you pass this test. A result less than 22 inches indicates a lack of strength. Exercises and programs to improve your strength base will help you achieve a higher vertical jump.

Mobility

Thoracic mobility is often overlooked. To test mobility, lie on your side with your knees bent in front of your body, nearly perpendicular to your hips (see figure 2.2). Open your chest, and as you twist your torso, reach your top arm behind you, attempting to lay your shoulder blades and the back of your hand on the floor. Test both sides. If you can accomplish this on both sides, it's a pass. If you fail either side, you should work on improving your mobility.

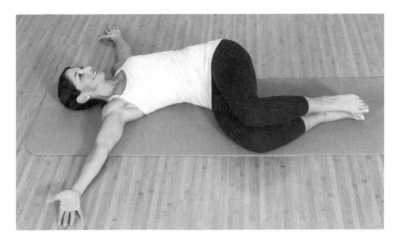

FIGURE 2.2 Thoracic mobility test.

Stability

Standing on one leg, bend the other knee and lift the leg off the ground until your thigh is parallel to the floor (see figure 2.3). Are you able to instantly stabilize and hold the position for at least 10 seconds, or do you have trouble remaining balanced? If so, where does the balance issue come from?

If you are able to stabilize without wobbling, you pass. If you immediately begin to fall over, you need to work on developing stability.

Agility

We do not recommend testing using the agility ladder because the patterns it uses are learned and therefore not neurologically driven. The pro shuttle drill is a better test to gauge how an athlete decelerates and accelerates out of cuts. This test is sometimes called the 5-10-5 drill and was made popular by the NFL Scouting Combine. Set three consecutive cones 5 yards (4.6 m) apart. Stand at the middle cone and

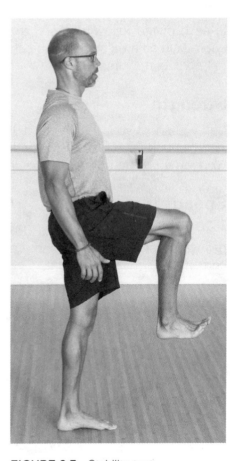

FIGURE 2.3 Stability test.

sprint to the next cone. Touch it before racing back past the center to the cone on the opposite end. At the third cone, come out of the cut and finish when you cross where you started at the middle cone.

Personal Assessment Record

Date: _____

Age: _____

Weight: _____

Resting heart rate: _____

Circumference Measurements

Chest: _____ Waist: _____ Hips: _____

Right biceps: _____ Left biceps: _____

Right thigh: _____ Left thigh: _____

Right calf: _____ Left calf: _____

Body Fat

Chest (men): _____

Triceps (women): _____

Abdominals (men): _____

Iliac crest (women): _____

Thigh: _____

Primary Assessments

Strength: _____

Speed: _____

Power: _____

Mobility: _____

Stability: _____

Agility: _____

Flexibility: _____

From A. Lademann and R. Lademann, *Pilates and Conditioning for Athletes: An Integrated Approach to Performance and Recovery* (Champaign, IL: Human Kinetics, 2019).

This drill shows whether athletes can keep their feet under them and maintain composure while decelerating and reaccelerating out of the cut. An acceptable time depends on the athlete and sport. Generally, less than 4.5 seconds is preferred.

Flexibility

One of easiest ways to assess your flexibility is with a **supine** hamstring test. Use a stretch strap or an 8-foot (2.4 m) yoga strap for this test. Start seated on the ground and loop the strap around the arch of one foot. Lie supine on the ground and raise that leg into the air, ideally to a 90-degree angle. If you can maintain your pelvic alignment without hiking one hip up or allowing your glutes and **sacrum** to lift off the floor, then you pass. If you must bend your knee to achieve a 90-degree angle or your glutes come off the floor, you fail and need to work on improving your flexibility.

Visualization Is Part of Goal Setting

Once you have identified your goal, the next step is visualization. Regardless of your sport, in order to achieve success and become healthier, stronger, faster, or more confident, you need a picture of your end goal in your mind.

To do this, create a detailed mental image of the desired outcome using all five of your senses. For example, if your goal is to run a marathon, visualize yourself in the event. Picture the starting line. See where you are running, notice the curves of the road and the smell and feel of the air. Taste the sweat as it passes over your lips. Feel your body moving with ease through the race. Be aware of the fans you're passing as they cheer you on. Notice the other racers you are passing. Feel all of your muscles working together; your body is in harmony and you're doing what you have been training to do. Imagine crossing the finishing line with your hands up in the air and a huge smile on your face. You look at your time and it's your personal best. You did it!

Playing this scene over and over in your mind and allowing your body to actually experience the race without leaving your chair is just as important as the physical portion of your conditioning. Treat your brain like a muscle: It needs to be trained as well as your body.

If using visualization is a new concept for you, know that it can work for anyone for just about any situation in life. The practice of visualization doesn't have to take long; it just needs to be done consistently. Even setting aside 5 to 10 minutes each day will help you reach your goals. We all have the power to visualize. Even though your goals haven't become reality, you can imagine that you have already achieved what you are working toward. So, once the big moment arrives, you've "done it" so many times before that you're ready to actually do it.

When visualizing your goals it is OK to also picture setbacks in order to devise plans for overcoming them. This may be beneficial so that you're not caught off guard when something unexpected occurs. Let's go back to the example of running a marathon. What if it begins to rain or you're feeling tired on race day? When factors could keep you from feeling or doing your best physically, it sets up a battle of wills. Reaching your goal becomes more of a mind game than a body game. Therefore, play out the what-ifs in your mind beforehand and establish a plan to circumvent the situation. For instance, you could react to the rain during your marathon by zoning inward and using it as fuel to run faster and get out of the rain.

Pam is a client of ours and a highly experienced marathoner who runs in races all over the world. She has run in a variety of weather conditions and with a multitude of injuries. She completed the 2018 Boston Marathon and, as you may know, it was cold, windy, and pouring rain. Not only did she complete the race, but she beat her previous time. When we asked her how she did it, she said it was her focus and mindset along with the cheering crowd down Boylston Street that kept her motivated to keep going.

Next Steps

At this point you have created your goal, assessed your body, and begun to visualize achieving your goal. Now your secondary assessments and body-work come in to the picture. How is your posture? Is it helping or hindering your overall performance? How large is your lung capacity? Are you using your breath to your advantage? How tight do you feel? Can you easily bend down while keeping your knees straight and set your palms on the floor? Do your joints feel open or locked up?

Do you move with ease, or is your movement heavy? In chapter 3, you will learn a variety of techniques that will assist in creating greater range of motion, fluidity, and flexibility through your entire body. You will be able to use techniques such as joint articulation and myofascial release daily to help you become a more fluid and in-control athlete.

3 | Daily Movements That Enhance Performance

Optimal athletic performance requires body awareness, an understanding of movement, and how to assess it. It's important to connect a physical movement with cognitive understanding. The best athletes don't perform movement just to move. They understand the process of the movement and embrace the process both physically and mentally.

Throughout this chapter you will learn warm-up and recovery techniques and tips you may use daily. Exercises and movement series will not only enhance your training capacity, but more importantly, your ability to recover. These techniques may be used before and after training, or you can use some of them on your recovery days.

The best athletes know not only how to commit to their training, but also how to commit to their recovery. They know how important taking time to fine-tune even the smallest detail is to their overall performance. Remember that it's not a single big effort that makes the largest impact; it's all the small things that happen along the way that affect your performance the most.

When people arrive at our facility for their sessions, most of them follow a similar warm-up protocol. It is vital that before you begin training, your body is warm and ready to go. This warm-up includes using the foam roller, performing the dynamic warm-up exercises, and checking your range of motion using the joint articulation series.

Align Yourself: How Important Is Your Posture?

Stand up straight. We have all heard it before, but what does it actually mean to be straight? Most of us know good posture when we see it and may be inspired by how free and strong it makes someone look regardless of age, size, or fitness level. And whether you're aware of it or not, we make judgments about other people, their athleticism, and their overall health and well-being by observing their posture.

Take a look around you and see how many people look down while they walk. They may be paying attention to their phones or the ground. Notice the position of their head, shoulders, and upper back. Is their gait easy and smooth? Are they shuffling their feet? Do they look strong, athletic, young, and fit? Or do they look tired, old, or lethargic?

Now look at someone who is walking tall. Their eyes are cast forward, their posture is straight, and their gait is easy and smooth. They seem to have an air about them and walk with confidence and ease. They may appear fit, strong, young, and athletic regardless of their age or size. Without even realizing it, you may be allowing your posture to hinder not only how you feel, but also your performance levels and how others perceive you.

The spine is made up of 24 moving vertebrae and about 9 fused vertebrae (see figure 3.1). (This number varies based on the fused vertebrae in the sacral and coccyx regions.) The spine is both strong and mobile. It should be able to twist, turn, and bend both forward and backward easily and without pain or tightness. In Pilates, we often talk about the pelvis and lower spine (known as the pelvic–lumbar region) because this is the area referred to as the powerhouse (core), where all movement is initiated.

Stabilizing your spine and working to create proper posture begins at the **pelvic floor**. Recruitment of these muscles should always be one of the first

Benefits of Proper Posture

- Keeps bones and joints in the correct alignment so that muscles are used properly
- Decreases abnormal wear on joints
- Decreases the stress on the ligaments in the spine
- Prevents the spine from becoming fixed, allowing it to move freely
- Requires less energy and helps to prevent fatigue
- Prevents backache and muscular pain
- Relies on the deep core muscles of the powerhouse (abdominals, back, and pelvic floor) to support proper posture; allows the shoulders to relax, the neck and head to move freely, and relieves stress on the hips, legs, and feet
- Contributes to a younger, healthier, longer, and leaner appearance

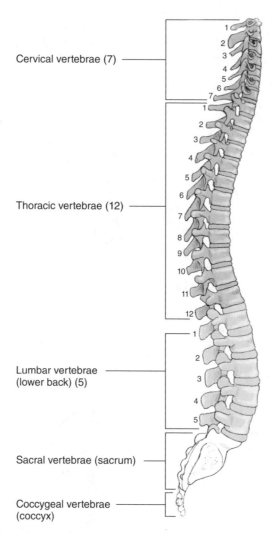

Cervical vertebrae (7)

Thoracic vertebrae (12)

Lumbar vertebrae
(lower back) (5)

Sacral vertebrae (sacrum)

Coccygeal vertebrae
(coccyx)

FIGURE 3.1 Lateral view of a healthy spine.

steps when engaging your powerhouse. Fortunately, because of how the body is designed, when the **transverse abdominal** muscles contract, so do the muscles of the pelvic floor. Pilates trains us to develop and use core strength rather than initiating movement with only the superficial muscles.

The pelvis is bowl shaped and made up of three bones: the ischium, ilium, and pubis (see figure 3.2). The **sacroiliac joint** is at the back of the pelvis. If the pelvis is misaligned, it could adversely affect movements up and down the body, resulting in inefficient movement, muscular imbalances, and stress on the rest of the body. If the pelvis is out of alignment, the rest of the spine will be as well. Detecting the imbalances is the first step; working to fix them is next.

Remember these cues for standing up straight as you begin your movement. Keeping the length of your spine, known as **axial elongation**, and the width of your shoulders in an ideal alignment will help you make the most of each movement (see figure 3.3).

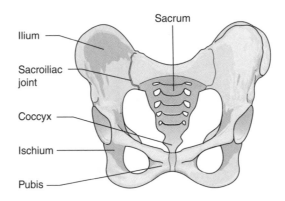

FIGURE 3.2   Frontal view of the pelvis.

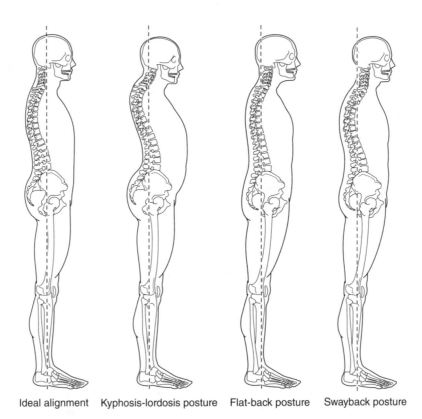

Ideal alignment   Kyphosis-lordosis posture   Flat-back posture   Swayback posture

FIGURE 3.3   Lateral view of ideal standing posture and common posture misalignments.

Check Your Posture

Find a room with a full-length mirror for this exercise.

1. Walk around the room to loosen your body, stopping in front of the mirror. Turn to one side.

2. Look at your feet and make sure they are in a parallel position about hip-distance apart, with equal weight from toe to heel and from the right to left side of each foot. You should feel like you're trying to push the floor away from you with your feet.

3. Feel your tailbone reaching down to the floor as if it were an extension cord you're trying to plug in. Your hamstrings should begin to engage. Knees are straight (not locked or hyperextended), and your **lumbar spine** should feel long.

4. Your torso should feel a bit forward as if you're leaning slightly in front of your pelvis. This will help your **rectus abdominis** muscles to engage.

5. Your arms should hang long by your sides, reaching your ring finger toward the floor as if it's your longest finger. As you do this, notice your shoulders relax and move down away from your ears.

6. The tips of your shoulders and width of your clavicles (collar bones) should feel wide and equal from the front to the back of your body. Make sure your shoulder blades are not pinching toward one another.

7. Your eyes should look straight ahead, with the crown of your head reaching toward the sky. The back of your head at the occipital ridge (where the skull meets the spine) should feel aligned with your upper back while your earlobes rest over (not in front of) your clavicles.

8. Notice the length of your spine and width across your chest. You should feel longer and more grounded, and the messages from your feet, hamstrings, and rectus abdominis should tell you that they are working to support you.

9. Your breathing should feel more active and easier, and you should be able to take longer, fuller breaths.

Breathing Techniques

Breathing sounds simple, right? We all do it, but how often do you actually think about how to breathe? People who have asthma or chronic obstructive pulmonary disease (COPD) think about breathing quite often. And if you have allergies or a cold, you may have difficulty breathing as well.

Has anyone ever told you to "just breathe" when they see that you're tired or stressed? Ever notice that by taking a long, deep breath, you can feel your body become more relaxed as you exhale? Breath is everything and is the one thing we all must do in order to live. But do you ever think about breathing in relationship to your movement or what style of breathing is most beneficial for what you're trying to accomplish?

There are numerous styles of breathing: nose-only breathing, mouth-only breathing, breathing through both the nose and mouth, breathing into the belly, and breathing into the diaphragm. You can practice breathing in yoga, for meditation and relaxation, for holding your breath if you're underwater, and so on. What you will learn is how to use your breath to your advantage. You will be able to increase not only your brain and body awareness and decrease your stress levels, but also how to harness your power, increase your endurance, and improve your overall performance levels by breathing correctly.

Belly Breathing

If you have taken a yoga class or tried meditation, then you have heard the benefits of breathing deeply into your belly. And for those purposes, it is a great way to relax, and "fill yourself with air." However, it is an incorrect way to breathe during Pilates or any movement that requires you to maintain your core strength and power.

In the book *Return to Life Through Contrology,* Joseph Pilates wrote that, "Breathing is the first act of life, and the last . . . . Above all, learn how to breathe correctly" (Pilates, 23). Breathing uses numerous muscles that contribute to your ability to inhale and exhale. The diaphragm is the most significant muscle used in breathing. It is large and dome shaped and is located at the base of the lungs. Your abdominal muscles help move the diaphragm and give you more power to empty your lungs. When the abdominal muscles are relaxed, they are allowed to push outward. Diaphragmatic, or belly, breathing is perfect for mediation and relaxation, but this form of breathing does not create the greatest amount of stability during movements.

Benefits of Breathing Correctly

- Oxygenates the blood and nourishes the body at a cellular level
- Calms the body and mind, reducing stress and anxiety
- Eliminates toxins from the body
- Improves circulation and skin clarity
- Creates a deeper connection to your core (powerhouse)
- Creates smooth movement patterns when movement and breathing patterns coincide

Lateral Breathing

Lateral breathing, otherwise known as intercostal breathing, emphasizes the lateral expansion of the rib cage while maintaining a consistent inward pull of the deep abdominal muscles during both your inhalation and exhalation. During lateral breathing, you inhale through your nose and exhale through

Practicing Belly Breathing and Lateral Breathing

Belly Breathing

1. Lie on your back with your knees bent and feet in a parallel position flat on the floor about hip-distance apart.

2. To begin, place one hand on your upper chest and your other hand on your belly button. Notice how much of your back is in contact with the floor. Feel your shoulder blades, your ribs, lower back, and glutes. Feel the equal weight on your upper and lower back and on the right and left side of your body.

3. As you inhale through your nose, allow your breath to travel deeply into your belly. Notice the rise of your belly as if you were filling a balloon. As you exhale through your mouth as if you were fogging up a mirror to leave someone a message, notice the air travel back out of your belly.

4. As you repeat the sequence, notice whether your lower back begins to lift away from the floor, creating a small arch. This limits your stability and control during movement.

Lateral Breathing

1. While in the same position as described for belly breathing, change the placement of your hands to the outside of your lower ribs. Again notice the back of your body and the connection you have to the floor.

2. Inhale through your nose. As you exhale through your mouth, draw your navel back toward your spine and imagine that it were glued there. As you begin to inhale again, imagine breathing into your side body as if you were a fish breathing into your gills. As you exhale through your mouth and "fog up the mirror," feel the ribs begin to knit together and move down toward your waist.

3. Repeat the exercise, this time paying attention to your back and the connection you have to the floor. You should feel just as connected during your inhalation as your exhalation.

When you become adept at both styles of breathing, you will be able to vary the location of your breath from belly to ribs as often as you choose.

your mouth. The exhale should allow the mouth to open as if you were fogging up a mirror to leave someone a message. The sound of the exhale is slightly audible and the jaw is relaxed and allowed to hang open slightly. During the exhalation, the lips should not be pursed as if you were blowing out a candle. This could create stress in your neck and throat.

The main reason to use lateral breathing is to help maintain the abdominal contraction while performing Pilates and other exercises. It's the ideal breathing technique for keeping a stable core and strong back, which are important for successful performance and for protecting the body. During the exhalation phase of Pilates and other exercises, the abdominal muscles contract, further assisting the diaphragm and intercostals in expelling air. This by no means implies that belly breathing is incorrect, only that lateral breathing is preferred for Pilates and other forms of movement that require coordination between breath and stability. Using lateral breathing with consistent engagement of the abdominals allows you to maintain a deeper abdominal contraction during both the inhalation and exhalation. This helps prepare the body for movement and exercise while also protecting the muscles of the back and around the spine. When practicing lateral breathing, inhale as you expand and lengthen the body, and exhale as you pull the body in toward its center.

Maintaining lateral breathing during movement may be challenging in the beginning, but once you learn the technique, you will see significant gains in your power and control. Having taught the technique for many years,

Rick's Tip

One of the golfers I coached was a competitive player on the PGA Tour. The player had worked with many performance coaches trying to find one that not only understood golf and conditioning, but his mindset as well. He understood that golf is a sport that requires a multitude of strengths if one is to be a successful competitor. Because the golfer was already in tune with his body, we started his training with a simple breathing technique. I taught him how to regulate his nervous system just by controlling his breathing. For this technique, he inhaled through his nose for 5 seconds and exhaled through his mouth for 5 seconds. I wanted him to practice this technique regularly during his next practice round and report his results. He came in for his next session a few days later and commented, "It's amazing that just through breath, I can control my stress or anxiety about a shot or hole." He said that using this approach allowed him to be present and stay connected to the game more. I was thrilled because it told me that the golfer was not only motivated to get better, but he was willing to change some things he had been doing for a long time.

As performance coaches, our job is to see the field, court, or course through our athletes' eyes. To do this, they have to let you into their world, and the golfer was certainly going to allow this. During his next session, we went over tissue and how important tissue care is. I explained that tight muscles don't shoot 68s. The name of the game is fluidity, specifically through the hips and thoracic spine. He understood this and realized how much he needed to address his self-care.

With this athlete, I went right to the jugular first. He was either going to get it or not, and it was going to be quick. We've found through the years there are two ways to do things: the right way and the wrong way. We're only interested in athletes who want to do it the right way. If you are going to invest your time with someone, even if they are paying you, make sure you are both working toward the same goals and agree on how to reach them. If not, move on. We guarantee your stress levels will be lessened dramatically.

the changes reported by athletes are notable. Whether your goal is bench-pressing more weight, cycling longer, or running marathons with greater ease and at a faster pace, learning this technique will offer your body an entirely new level of performance.

Myofascial Release

When you bend forward, can you place your hands flat on the floor, or do they stop somewhere near your knees? When you sit on the floor with your legs fully extended in front of you, are you able to sit tall without feeling a grip in your hamstrings or low back, or do you slump or lean? When you stand in a doorframe with your back against the jamb and feet slightly in front of you, are your back and head against the jamb or do they pull forward? These are tests that determine how tight your muscles might be.

An effective way to eliminate pain and tightness and restore greater mobility is through myofascial release. What is myofascial release? It is a safe and effective technique for applying mild and slow sustained pressure into the fascia, the band of connective tissue beneath the skin that attaches, stabilizes, encloses, and separates muscle. When the fascia is tight, muscles are unable to perform as they should and the likelihood of an injury is greater. A variety of techniques will release the fascia. Techniques such as active release therapy and massage therapy are performed by a practitioner. Self-care techniques include foam rollers and other myofascial release tools. The best athletes have the most responsive tissue, meaning that although they may become sore and tight, their tissue responds almost immediately to myofascial release and becomes moveable, softer, and ready for the next workout.

Athletes must pay attention to the quality of their tissue. Tissue that is supple moves in a fluid state. Tissue that is fibrotic and hard tends to move in a less fluid state. To be a good mover, you need good tissue! Because most athletes don't have a massage therapist available often, it's crucial that they understand how to treat their own tissue.

Foam rolling, lacrosse ball therapy, and manual self-therapy are myofascial release techniques athletes can practice on themselves. When working on a problem area, you'll find a point where the pain originates, called a hot spot. Many people will avoid working on this point in the body, but this is the area you should focus on. Tissue responds to pressure, so apply direct pressure to the hot spot until the pain subsides. For example, if you are rolling out your **iliotibial band**, don't be tempted to roll quickly over the most painful areas. This can be difficult, but it will yield results. Prolonged pressure will soften the tissue and allow it to become reactive.

The tighter the muscles, the more pain and discomfort you may feel throughout your body. Often, the few minutes of stretching most people do before or after a workout isn't enough to release muscles and prevent injury.

And most people don't consider having a massage or body work done until they are unable to move. This is where your foam roller comes into play. Use it daily as part of your fitness routine.

Foam Rolling

Even the toughest athletes cringe when they think about foam rolling. If you haven't added foam rolling to your exercise routine, start now! A rolling program will increase your flexibility, range of motion, and so much more. When you use a foam roller, keep these tips in mind.

- Use a traditional smooth-surfaced roller that is 36 inches (91 cm) by 3 inches (8 cm).

- When you find the trigger point or hot spot, hold it until the area softens. Make sure you continue to breathe!

- Roll slowly over the area a few times; it may not relax on the first try.

- Keep it slow. Release work is done slowly; do not make quick, short moves.

- You're looking for a release of the muscle tissue. For some people that could take a minute or two and be five rolls. Others may need to stay in one location for 5 minutes and take 30 rolls back and forth.

Foam rolling should be a regular part of your warm-up for every workout. The following sections describe proper execution of these movements.

Nervous System Activation

This activation is a great way to wake up your body and prepare for additional movement. It also feels awesome to release the tension in your head, neck, and shoulders.

Why Can Rolling Be Painful?

- The compression of the roller on the soft tissue breaks up the knots in your muscles.

- Often, the knot itself isn't the source of the pain, but when it is triggered, it sends pain signals elsewhere in the body.

- Holding your breath or breathing shallowly will cause your muscles to resist and become even tighter. Take deep breaths while rolling to help relax your muscles and release the knots.

The following position applies to the head tilt and head nod exercises.

1. Place a foam roller lengthwise on the floor and lie supine (faceup) on it so your head and tailbone both rest on the roller.
2. Your feet are flat on the floor about hip-distance apart, your knees and feet are aligned, and your feet remain on the floor.

HEAD TILT

Complete the head tilt before doing additional opening exercises. It is ideal for releasing tension, strain, and tightness in your trapezius and neck and the base of your skull.

TECHNIQUE

1. Make sure the occipital ridge (base of your skull) is on the edge of the roller.
2. Apply as much pressure as tolerable as you turn your head from one side to the other as if you were saying "no." Move slowly and keep your eyes open.

REPETITION

Complete three to five times to each side.

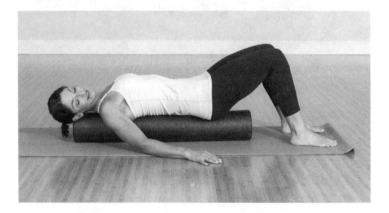

HEAD NOD

The head nod, like the head tilt, should be completed before additional opening exercises. It is also ideal for releasing tension, strain, and tightness in your trapezius and neck and the base of your skull.

TECHNIQUE

1. Rest the occipital ridge (base of your skull) on the edge of the roller.
2. Nod your head backward and forward as if you were saying "yes."
3. Apply as much pressure at the occipital ridge as possible as you nod your head up and down.
4. Move slowly and deliberately.

REPETITION

Complete three to five times in each direction.

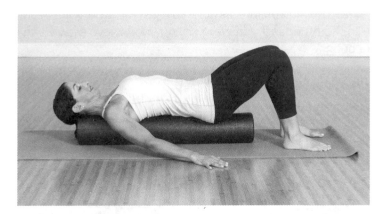

SHOULDER ROLL

While some people carry their stress from life in their head and neck, others feel the strain and pain in their shoulders. The shoulder roll is ideal for releasing the tension in your traps, rhomboids, and scapulae. You may feel the release in other areas as well.

TECHNIQUE

1. Lie supine on the roller, resting your head and tailbone on the roller.
2. Knees are bent and feet are flat on the floor.
3. Extend your arms to the side walls with the palms facing upward and breathe into the stretch for about three to five breath cycles (a).

4. Place your palms on the floor about 45 degrees away from your body *(b)*.

5. Roll from shoulder blade to shoulder blade slowly.

6. You will notice your hips sliding slightly off the roller as your body shifts. Return to center after each side.

REPETITION

Complete three to five times to each side.

TIP

If you feel a knot anywhere, remain on that spot and breathe deeply until you feel the knot release.

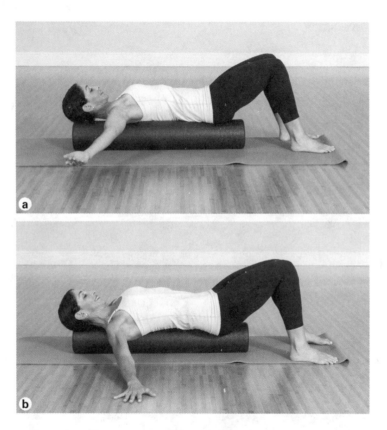

CHEST OPENER

Tightness in either your chest, shoulders, or upper back frequently contributes to tightness in the other two areas. Typically, if your back is tight so is your chest. For proper breathing, posture, and athletic performance, it's important that your chest be not only strong, but also open and relaxed to prevent postural imbalances and excessive kyphosis (an exaggerated forward rounding of the back).

TECHNIQUE

1. Lie faceup on the roller, resting your head and tailbone on the roller.
2. Knees are bent and feet are flat on the floor.
3. Bring arms to 90 degrees so that your wrist, elbow, and shoulder are in a straight line *(a)*.
4. Palms face in toward each other.
5. Inhale as you open your arms out to the width of your shoulders and they float about 5 inches (13 cm) above the floor *(b)*.
6. Exhale as you bring your arms back to the starting place.

REPETITION

Complete five times.

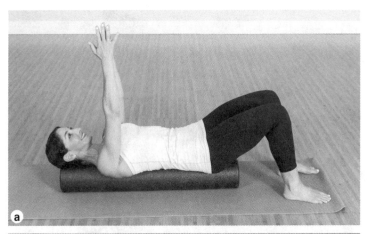

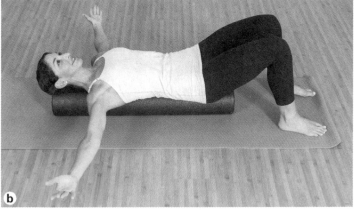

HIP ROLL

Many people with tight hip flexors and glutes complain of lower-back tightness or pain. By working to stabilize your pelvis and open your hip flexors, you can release some of the tension and strain throughout your lower back.

TECHNIQUE

1. Lie supine on the roller. Knees are bent and feet are flat on the floor.
2. Palms are 45 degrees away from body on the floor.
3. Inhale as the leg rolls open and extends away from the hip, lengthening away from the body *(a and b)*. Exhale to return to starting position.

REPETITION

Repeat two times in each direction and then change legs.

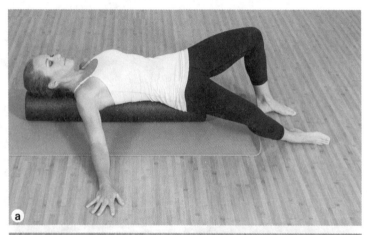

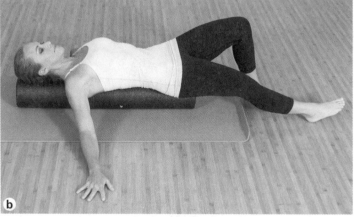

SIDE STRETCH WITH LOW LUNGE

This exercise opens the ribs and works the psoas, hip flexor, and thigh.

TECHNIQUE

1. Come into a low lunge with your back knee on the floor.
2. Hold the roller at each end in front of you.
3. Raise the roller directly over your head while maintaining straight arms.
4. Inhale to bend to the side and exhale to return to center *(a and b)*.

REPETITION

Bend to each side three to five times, and then lunge on the other leg.

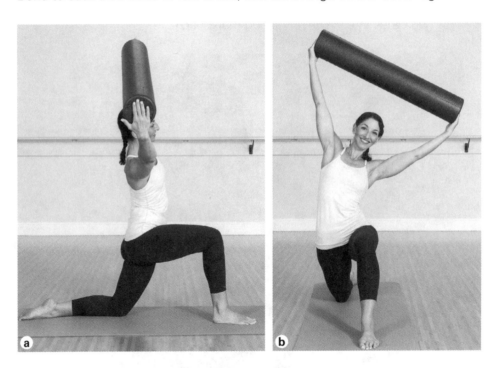

PIRIFORMIS STRETCH

A daily **piriformis** stretch is a must for just about everyone. The piriformis is a small muscle located deep within the glutes that starts at the lower back and connects to the thigh bone (femur). Opening your hips and releasing your glutes and piriformis will increase your depth in a squat, lengthen your running stride, and develop overall better movement patterns.

TECHNIQUE

1. Sit on the floor and place the foam roller horizontally in front of you.
2. Place one shin bone across the roller, working to bring your knee and ankle on top of the roller and maintaining your hips forward.
3. Extend your back leg as straight as you can behind you, and rest the top of your thigh on the floor. If you are able, press your heel to the back wall to lift your thigh above the floor, which may increase your stretch.
4. Hands remain shoulder-width apart either on the roller or on the floor in front of the roller.
5. Inhale to fold forward and remain there for five breaths.
6. Return to the starting position and change sides.

REPETITION

Three to five breaths on each side is perfect. No repetitions.

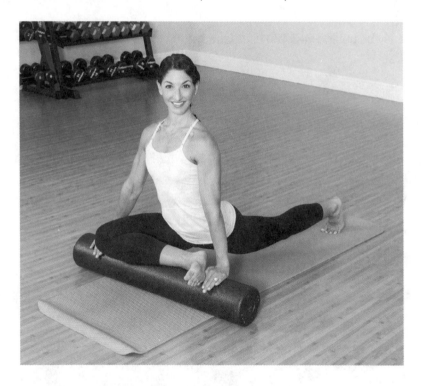

Rolling Series

When rolling out your body, the movements should be smooth and slow and use a full range of motion. Think of painting a wall using long, even strokes instead of short choppy ones.

SUPINE BACK ROLL

The supine back roll, otherwise known as the back massage, is most people's favorite roll. You can start at your traps and roll as low as your waistband.

TECHNIQUE

1. Place the roller on the floor, and lie back on it so it is under your shoulder blades. Your head should be higher than your hips, and your glutes should be a few inches above the floor *(a)*.
2. The feet are flat and knees bent.
3. Push and pull with your feet to create movement as you roll from the top of your shoulder to your waistband *(b)*.
4. Repeat until you feel a release in your back muscles. If you're counting, try rolling down and back up 4 to 10 times.

TIP

Hands may be behind your head, crossed at the chest, or extended to the sides.

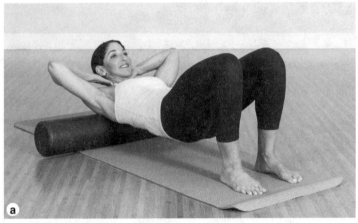

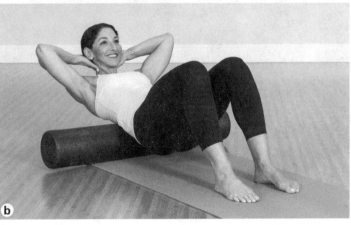

GLUTE RELEASE

Tight glutes—most of us have them—can lead to a host of other issues and compensations. A variety of techniques will release all areas of your glutes; this one is the best for rolling out your gluteus maximus, minimus, and medius.

TECHNIQUE

1. Begin by sitting on the roller. Knees are bent and feet are flat on the floor.
2. One hand is on the floor at your side. The other hand may be on your lap or the opposite knee *(a)*. Begin rolling slowly from the outside of the hip and down one glute *(b)*.
3. You can roll from your waistband to the base of your glutes.

REPETITION

Roll each side at least five times slowly.

VARIATION

Cross one ankle over the other knee as if you're sitting in a chair.

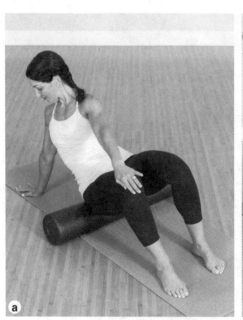
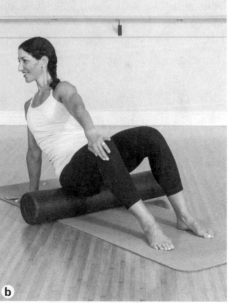

HAMSTRING STRETCH

This hamstring stretch reminds us of trying to squeeze the last bit of toothpaste out of the tube. Think of it as more of a hold stretch while using your breath to release the tension and tightness in your hamstrings than a rolling technique. Tight hamstrings may send the sensation up to your glutes and low back or down to your feet. In either case, additional pain and tightness may occur.

TECHNIQUE

1. Begin by sitting on the roller with legs extended in front of you.
2. Bend one knee, keeping your foot flat on the floor.
3. Rotate your body and reach your opposite hand toward the straight leg or toes. Your other hand remains on the floor to assist with stability *(a)*.
4. Roll the roller slightly down past the lower part of your glutes, hold, and breathe. After a few breath cycles, roll the roller farther down your hamstring, remaining still for at least three breaths before moving the roller lower toward the back of your knee *(b)*.

REPETITION

Repeat the sequence on the other side.

TIP

This is an intense stretch, so move slowly and be sure to breathe.

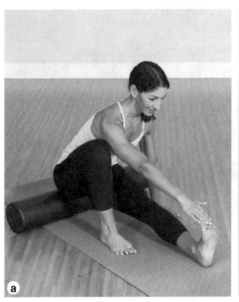
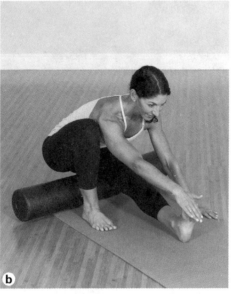

CALF STRETCH

Many of us rely on a traditional stretch at the wall to release our calf muscles. This rolling sequence is an important add-on and should be performed often. Tight calf muscles may contribute to poor stride length when running and limited response time and shorter lateral moves in sports such as tennis and pickleball.

TECHNIQUE

1. Sit on the floor with both knees bent and the roller under your knees. Bring one foot toward you behind the roller, keeping your foot flat on the floor. Straighten the other leg over the roller, maintaining a flexed foot position.
2. Palms are flat on the floor behind you for balance and support.
3. Lift your body off the floor and roll the roller from the back of your knee *(a)* to your ankle *(b)*.
4. Roll slowly and rotate your foot and leg internally and externally to release your entire calf.

REPETITION

Repeat five to eight times and repeat on the other leg.

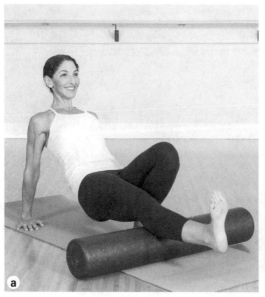
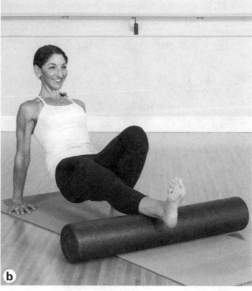

IT BAND RELEASE

Found on the outside of your leg, between your hip and the outside of your knee, your IT band may be the cause of knee and low-back issues. When the IT band is tight, everything is tight, and it may contribute to a feeling of pulling in your knee and to gait and hip issues.

TECHNIQUE

1. Lie on your side with your body in a straight line, and place the roller between your hip and knee *(a)*. The movement will follow the seam of your pants.
2. Hands or forearms are on the floor.
3. Roll from your waistband down to the knee *(b)*.
4. Move slowly, keeping the rolling action long and smooth. If you feel a knot, allow your body to remain on top of it and breathe until you feel a slight release.

REPETITION

Repeat the sequence on the other side.

TIP

For less resistance, bend your top leg at the knee and place your foot flat on the floor in front of you. Extending and stacking both legs creates more pressure.

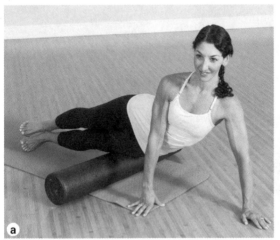
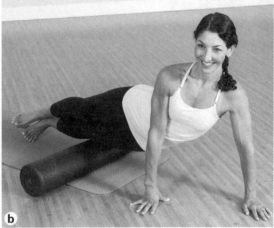

QUADRICEPS RELEASE

When rolling your quadriceps, start at your hip flexor and roll down to your kneecap in long strokes. Roll one leg at a time to get the full benefit. Because a variety of muscles work together within your quads, you can miss areas when both thighs are on top of the roller at the same time. By rolling one leg at a time, you can rotate both internally and externally to release all the way up to your hip flexors.

TECHNIQUE

1. Support yourself on your hands and knees and place the foam roller under you horizontally.
2. With your palms on the floor under your shoulders, lower your body so that your thigh rests on the roller.
3. Move your other leg to the side and bend that knee toward your elbow *(a)*.
4. Use your palms on the floor to assist in rolling the thigh from your hip flexor to the top of your knee *(b)*. Avoid rolling over your patella.

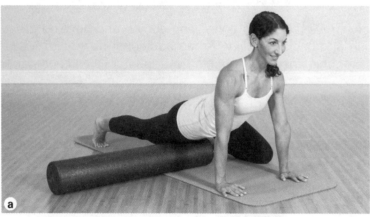

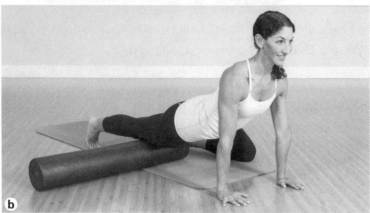

REPETITION

Roll slowly until you feel the fascia begin to release, or at least 4 to 10 times.

TIPS

- If there is too much pressure on your hands and wrists, place your forearms on the floor instead.
- Roll your entire quad by rotating slightly inward and outward.
- Roll slowly using long, even strokes.

Now that your body is warm, you're ready to begin your foam roller workout. The following exercises might be challenging whether you're new to them or a veteran athlete. Each movement requires use of the Pilates principles: breath, centering, concentration, control, flow, and precision. You will need to connect your breath to your movement in order to find your balance and stability for each exercise.

Articulation Exercises

The following exercises are done lying supine and develop greater spinal articulation and back flexibility. As an additional benefit of lying over the foam roller in this position is opening your pectorals and anterior deltoids.

BRIDGE

This exercise activates the spine. The segmental movement increases range of motion.

TECHNIQUE

1. Lie on the roller so that your head and tailbone rest on it.
2. The knees are bent and feet are flat on the floor about hip-distance apart.
3. Palms are 45 degrees away from body and flat on the floor.
4. Inhale as you tip your pubic bone slightly up toward the sky, creating a slight scoop of the lower abdominals *(a)*.
5. Exhale as you raise your pelvis and begin to peel your spine off the roller one vertebra at a time until you reach the tip of your shoulder blades *(b)*.

REPETITION

Repeat four times.

TIP

The pubic bone should remain higher than your rib cage so that you maintain your pelvic tilt.

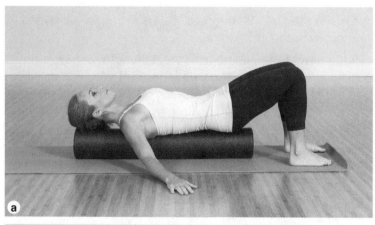

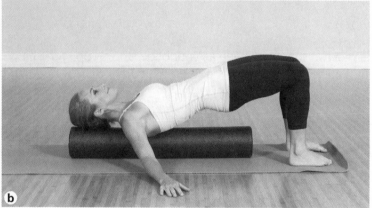

AB CURL

This exercise strengthens the core, works flexion, and activates the pelvic floor.

TECHNIQUE

1. Lie on the roller with the head and entire spine resting on it.
2. The knees are bent and feet are flat on the floor, hip-distance apart.
3. Arms are in the air at 90 degrees, palms facing forward, and thumbs in alignment with the armpits *(a)*.
4. Draw the navel to the spine, and create length at your lumbar spine by reaching your tailbone to the wall in front of you. This creates a scooping of the abdominals. Keep the back of your ribs and spine in contact with the roller.
5. Slightly tuck your chin toward your chest so that your eyes gaze forward toward your knees. Inhale to prepare and exhale to peel your upper body off the roller to the tip of your shoulder blades *(b)*.

REPETITION

Repeat up to 10 times.

TIP

Your arms move at the same pace as your body, ending up at the height of your hips about 3 inches (8 cm) from the floor.

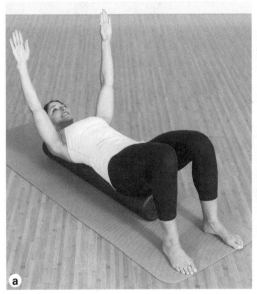
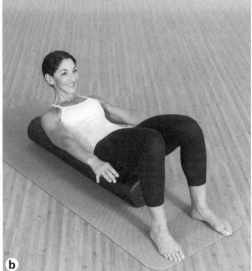

Core Stability and Control Exercises

When we talk about your core, we are not discussing only your rectus abdominis (six-pack), we mean your entire powerhouse. Doing the following exercises on the roller not only works the specific area that the exercise targets, but it also stabilizes your pelvis and works your entire powerhouse.

TOE TAP

This exercise works the **transverse abdominals**, **obliques**, and hip flexors and develops breath control.

TECHNIQUE

1. Lie faceup, with the knees bent. Feet are flat on the floor, hip-distance apart, and palms are flat on the floor, 45 degrees away from the body.

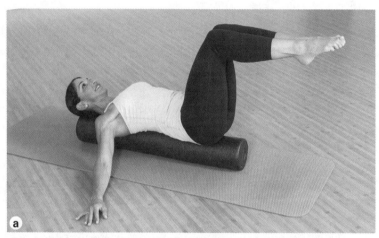

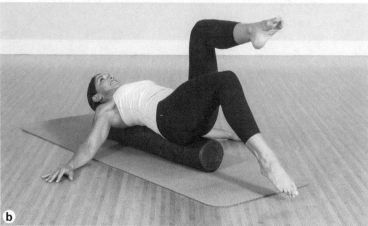

2. The chin is slightly tucked, and the eyes gaze forward.

3. Exhale to engage the core and create the scoop. Inhale to prepare, and while exhaling, take one foot off the floor at a time into a tabletop position *(a)*.

4. Inhale as you lower one leg from the hip and tap the toe on the floor *(b)*.

5. Exhale to return to the starting position.

REPETITION

Inhale and repeat four more times before switching sides.

LEG LOWER

This exercise works the transverse abdominals, obliques, and hip flexors and stretches the hamstrings and calves. It also develops breath control.

TECHNIQUE

1. Lie supine, keeping the knees bent and feet flat on the floor, hip-distance apart. The palms are flat on the floor, 45 degrees away from the body.

2. The chin is slightly tucked, and eyes gaze forward.

3. Exhale to engage the core and create a scoop. Inhale to prepare, and while exhaling, take one foot at a time off the floor into a tabletop position. Fully extend the legs toward the sky (90 degrees and shut together in a parallel position) while keeping the sacrum and tailbone in contact with the roller *(a)*.

4. Inhale as you lower your straight legs to the lowest point at which your back is in contact with the roller, core is engaged, neck is long, and eyes are forward *(b)*.

5. Exhale as you return your straight legs to the starting position.

REPETITION

Repeat 6 to 10 times.

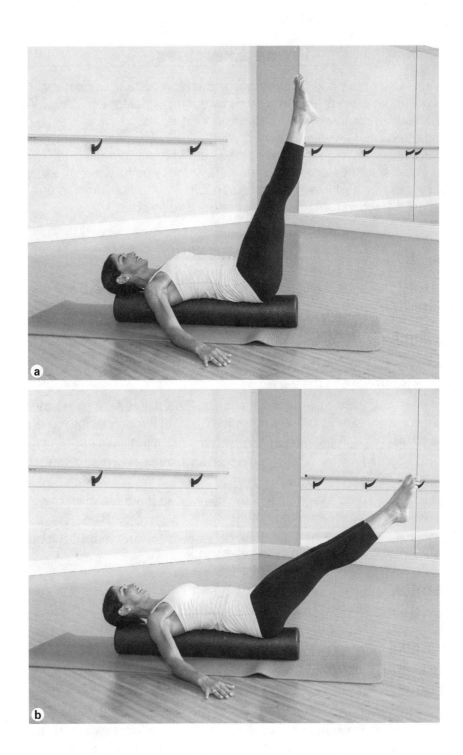

Prone Exercises

Working in a prone position stretches and strengthens your posterior chain (the back of your body, including the hamstrings, glutes, and back). When lying facedown or in a quadruped position, it is important to maintain the feeling of pulling your navel toward your spine and creating length in your lumbar spine. Many people are somewhat kyphotic, meaning their upper spine is excessively curved and their shoulders pull forward. A variety of exercises performed in a prone position can counteract this postural misalignment, which in turn improves strength and flexibility.

SHOULDER SHRUG

This exercise extends the upper thoracic spine, opens the chest, and releases the shoulders.

TECHNIQUE

1. Lie on your belly with legs extended behind you and your arms extended forward, close to the ears.
2. Place the foam roller under the wrists. The palms face each other and fingers are extended. The arms remain straight throughout the movement.
3. Tip the pelvic bone toward floor, pull the navel toward spine, and retract the shoulders by pulling the shoulder blades down and toward the spine *(a)*.
4. Inhale to shrug the shoulders to your ears as the foam roller moves forward away from your body *(b)*.
5. Exhale as you shrug your shoulders down toward your back pockets, while keeping the elbows straight.

REPETITION

Repeat five to eight times.

VARIATIONS

You may also do this exercise with one arm at a time.

1. Keep one arm flat on the floor at your side and repeat the exercise with the wrist of the other arm on the roller.
2. Your body stays still and you inhale to roll the foam roller forward and exhale as the foam roller comes back to the starting position.

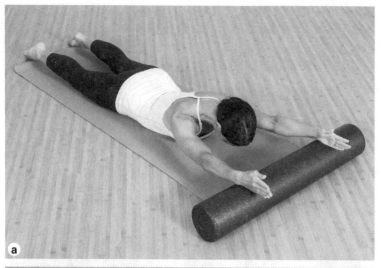

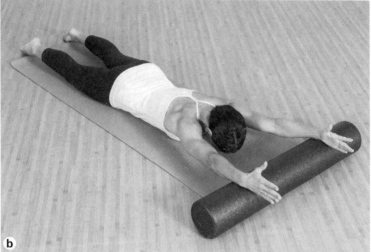

SWAN

During this extension from a prone position, you will feel a stretch through the length of your abdominals, an opening across your clavicles, and work in your middle back extensors.

TECHNIQUE

1. Lie on your belly, with legs extended behind you and your arms extended forward and close to your ears.

2. Place the foam roller under the wrists, with the palms facing each other and fingers extended. The arms remain straight throughout the movement.

3. Tip the pelvic bone toward the floor, draw the navel toward the spine, and pull the shoulders down toward your back pockets *(a)*.

4. As you inhale, peel your chest off the floor while maintaining proper head and neck alignment. Rise as high as you can without compromising form *(b)*. This is typically to the middle portion of the ribs. If you feel pinching or negative feedback at your low back near your waistband, you have risen too high off the floor.

5. Exhale to return to your starting position.

REPETITION

Repeat three to five times.

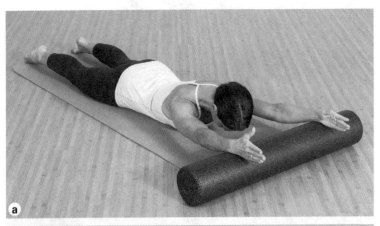

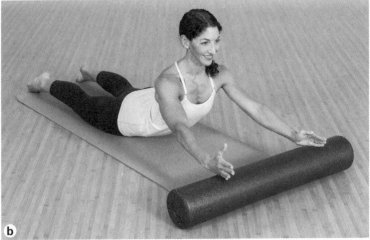

PLANK AND PUSH-UP SERIES

Planks are not only ideal for strengthening and stabilizing your shoulder girdle, but they also are great core exercises. The instability of the foam roller requires you to stabilize your plank in an entirely new way.

This exercise works the chest, core, upper back, arms, and shoulders.

TECHNIQUE

1. Hands are shoulder-width apart on the roller, with thumbs and fingers cupping the roller.
2. Legs are fully extended and heels reach toward the back wall *(a)*.
3. Remain in the plank position for 5 to 10 breath cycles. If you need a break prior to continuing into the push-up sequence, feel free to bring your knees to the floor. If you are able to execute the following push-up sequence, do so without a break.
4. To complete the push-up, inhale to lower the body toward the roller, which is aligned with your chest *(b)*.

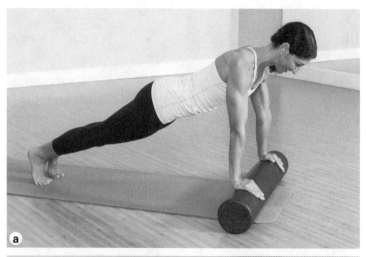

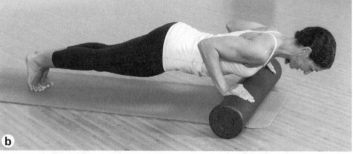

VARIATIONS

- To modify, bring knees to the floor, maintaining your body in a straight line from knees to shoulders during the plank and the push-up.
- For a more advanced option, place the balls of the feet on the roller and hands on the floor. Work to keep the roller still while holding the plank or doing the push-up.

Side Stretches

Lateral flexion not only opens the intercostal muscles, but depending on your position, it may also open and increase the sense of space in your psoas. Maintain proper form throughout the exercise to avoid twisting or putting torque on your spine during these movements.

MERMAID

This exercise opens the latissimus dorsi, stretches the hips, engages the obliques, stretches the spine, and increases breath control.

TECHNIQUE

1. Begin in a Z-sit position, with one shin bone in front of you and the other leg behind you, creating a Z with your legs. Distribute your weight equally on both sit bones *(a)*. If this position is uncomfortable, sit with legs crossed or straight.
2. The forearm is extended over the roller, fingers extended and palm facing forward. The foam roller should begin about 10 inches from your hips and extend away from the body as you straighten your bottom arm.
3. Inhale into lateral flexion *(b)*. Exhale to return to the starting position.

REPETITION

Repeat three times on each side.

TIP

The body should stay on the same plane throughout the movement.

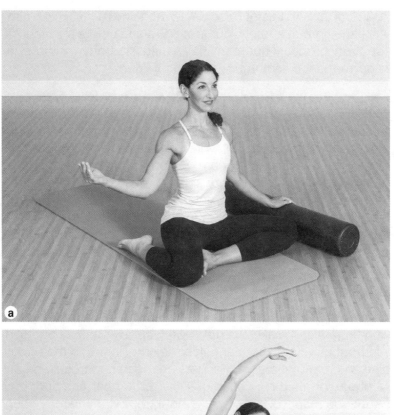

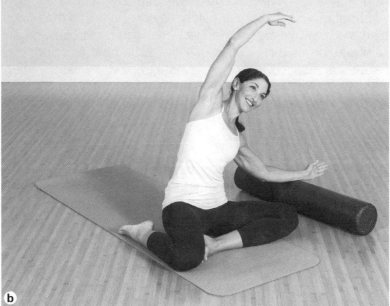

Open Your Joints

Thanks to Tim Adams of coachtimadams.com, this joint articulation series is used around the world. Many times, our bodies work in a state of compensation because of current or past injuries. Joint articulation exercises increase your range of motion and enhance your ability to move. For example, your foot is an important first point of contact when you move. How many times do you take the time to stretch your foot and ankle before an event? If you're like most of us, probably not many. Preparing the body for movement can improve performance and reduce the risk of injury.

Joint Articulation Series

The joint articulation series eliminates compensatory factors throughout the body while opening the joints, allowing for full range of motion. This series provides an effective pregame or preworkout routine and, when done consistently, allows for greater mobility and improved performance.

You will see significant improvement after doing some of the exercises in this series, while others will result in minimal or no improvement at all. The purpose of this series is to benefit your body so if any moves in this sequence reap no improvement, you can omit them from your articulation series.

Starting Position

To start the joint articulation series, stand tall with bare feet. Interlock your hands and fingers and make an arrow with your two index fingers, pointing directly in front of you at about shoulder height. Rotate to the right through your spine and mark where your fingers are pointing. It could be a spot on a wall, a photo, or anything you can easily remember and spot during the series. After you mark your spot to the right, repeat the same sequence on the left and mark your rotation point. You will begin the exercises with the ankle, an often-ignored joint.

Ankle Joint

Hold each position in each exercise for 15 to 20 seconds. The ankle is a hinge joint that creates dorsiflexion and plantar flexion. This joint is often overlooked in the broad scheme of training. It's important that we take time to address this joint since it's our first point of contact to the ground.

TOES UP

This is your first opportunity to address the ankle and make sure it moves correctly.

TECHNIQUE

1. Step back with your right foot so that your back knee has a slight bend to it.
2. Drive the big toe of your right foot down into the ground. You should feel a stretch in the bottom of your right foot, which may be more or less intense depending on your level of mobility.

3. Once you have pressed your big toe into the ground, internally rotate your foot to put pressure on the inside portion of your big toe.

4. Rotate the foot externally to drive all of your toes into the ground, with the emphasis on your two outermost toes.

REPETITION

Repeat the sequence with the other foot. Hold for three to five breath cycles.

TIP

If the pressure under your foot is uncomfortable, take pressure off your big toe until you feel comfortable with the stretch.

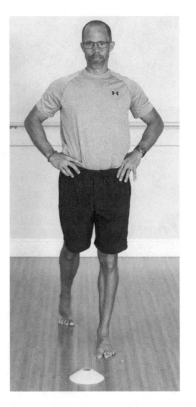

TOES DOWN

In this exercise, instead of driving the bottom of your foot down, you will drive the top of the foot toward the ground.

TECHNIQUE

1. Begin by taking a half step back and place the top of your foot and toes on the ground. Press your toes into the ground.

2. Rotate your ankle internally so that there is more pressure on the big-toe side of your foot; press down and hold.

3. Rotate the foot externally; press down and hold.

REPETITION

Repeat the sequence with the other foot. Hold each step of this technique for 3 to 5 breath cycles, about 20 seconds or so.

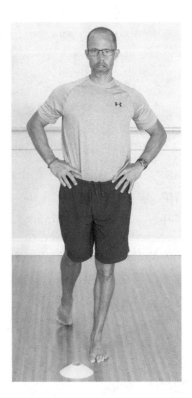

TIP

Once you have completed both sequences, use the following process to evaluate whether your articulation and mobility have improved.

1. Put your feet together, interlock your hands and feet, and point straight out.
2. Rotate to the right and compare your end point to your original marker to see whether there is significant improvement, minimal improvement, or no improvement at all.
3. Repeat on the left side and compare your result to your original mark.

Knees

Knee circles are a great way to warm up the knees and ankles simultaneously. Coordinating these two joints creates smoother movement.

KNEE CIRCLES

You might have done knee circles in gym class back in the day. They are a simple rotation of the knee and ankles that may have seemed silly back then, but they actually help to open your joints.

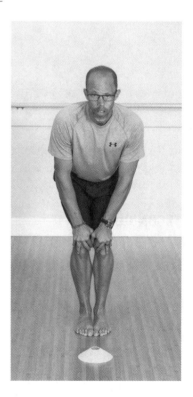

TECHNIQUE

1. Stand with your feet together and a slight bend in the knees, almost in a quarter-squat position.
2. Place your hands on your knees and make sure the knees are aligned over your toes.
3. Make 10 small clockwise circles with the knees, then make 10 in the other direction.

TIP

Once you have completed 10 circles in each direction, stand up and evaluate your articulation and mobility using the previously listed tip.

Hip Joints

The hip joint consists of a ball and socket that creates movement at the pelvis. The hips drive the knees, and the knees drive the ankles. At this point you should start to understand how energy is passed from one joint to the next to create movement. We want everyone to use the initial test system before moving onto the next joint area so that they understand the value of this sequence.

HIP CIRCLES

Hip circles use a basic rotation and feel great when you do them.

TECHNIQUE

1. Stand with your feet together and your hands on your hips. Bend the knees slightly to allow a greater range of motion.
2. Rotate your hips slowly clockwise, bending as far backward and forward as your body allows.

REPETITION

Complete 10 circles in each direction.

TIP

Make the movement big enough that you feel the stretch through your pelvic area, low back, and hip flexors.

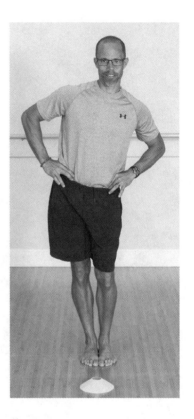

HIP FLEXION AND EXTENSION

Flexing and extending through the hips creates movement in your spine. Often, one movement feels better than the other, so feel free to repeat the movement that feels best.

TECHNIQUE

1. Stand with your feet together, place your hands on your hips, and bend forward, feeling a stretch in your posterior chain *(a)*.
2. Once you have reached the lowest point, slowly rise and extend backward until you reach your maximum range of motion *(b)*.

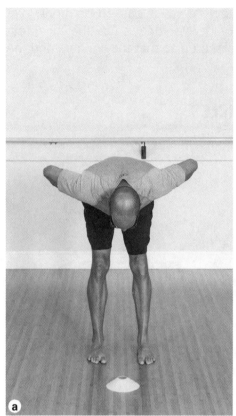 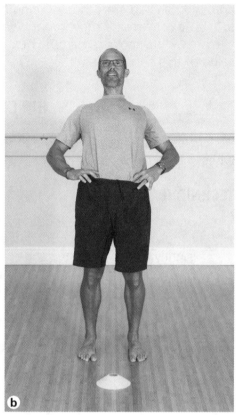

REPETITION

Complete 10 repetitions forward and backward. With each repetition, try to extend and flex a little more than the previous time to ensure you are fully reaching your mobility limits.

RETEST

Now that you have made your way through the ankle, knee, and hip joint openers, we want you to retest in order to evaluate how much progress you notice from just these first three joint openers.

HOW TO EVALUATE YOUR MOBILITY

Hold your arms straight out front, rotate both to your left and right. Compare your rotation outcome now to your initial rotation marks. If you see improvement, this is a positive. It tells you that you should keep these exercises in your articulation series. If there is no improvement, omit the hip exercises from your routine and continue on to the next joint, your neck.

Neck

The **cervical spine** and the structures around it need to be warm before a workout.

LATERAL FLEXION

Start by centering your head, then tilt your head from side to side, lowering your ear toward your shoulder on one side and then the other. This motion warms up the trapezius and scalenes.

REPETITION

Repeat three times on each side, holding each one for at least one to two full breath cycles.

CHIN EXTENSION AND FLEXION

This exercise looks a little strange, but give it your full attention and you'll be amazed by the extra movement it can create.

1. Place two fingers on your chin and push your chin and neck as far back as possible *(a)*.

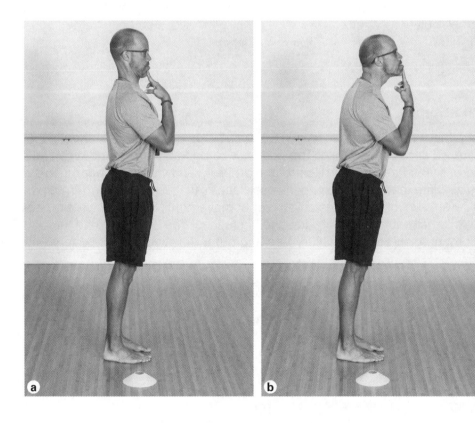

2. Move your chin straight back rather than down toward your chest.

3. Imagine a string running straight from your chin through the back of your head. Now slide your head back and forth along the string.

4. Extend your neck forward as far as possible, making sure your chin moves along a straight line and doesn't extend upward (b). Extend as far as your body allows.

REPETITION

Complete six repetitions.

TIP

Go back and do another retest to evaluate whether the neck exercise has a positive effect on your mobility. If it does, keep this move in your articulation series; if it has a minimal or no effect, omit it from your series.

The easiest way to remember which exercises have a positive effect is to write them down as you go. After you have completed the articulation series, you should feel more mobile and your joints should feel more open. You can conduct this series before any physical activity to ensure that you are not compensating and are fully ready to perform. Most of our athletes who play rotational sports (e.g., golf, tennis, pickleball, baseball, softball) notice huge differences in their overall mobility after completing the entire joint articulation series.

Used with permission of Coach Tim Adams, www.coachtimadams.com.

Next Steps

Now that you've completed our full warm-up, your muscles should feel activated and ready to train. The body is a remarkable thing, and when you address your posture, learn to breathe properly, and warm up your muscles, you alleviate the need for compensatory factors that can hinder performance. This warm-up routine will establish proper movement patterns. It's the collection of small habits that will add up to big results. The habits formed through this routine will keep you injury free and outperforming your opponent.

4 | Movement Prep: Dynamic Warm-Up

Gone are the days of the 5-minute warm-up consisting of a little jogging and some static stretches. We now know that optimal performance requires preparing the body's systems. To get an athlete ready for an upcoming session, we use a variety of warm-up techniques. A thorough warm-up may take 15 to 20 minutes if done correctly and awakens the nervous system, activates tissue, and raises core body temperature. Our base dynamic warm-up, featured in this chapter, is an example of a comprehensive warm-up. The length of the warm-up is affected by the age of the athlete and past or current injuries. Because, for example, player A may have arthritic knees, it may take them 30 minutes to get ready to squat. To develop an effective routine, you have to understand the process and work around limitations. It's been said that an effective warm-up can lower soft tissue injuries by 40 percent. Because of this, we teach athletes that it's important to carry your specific warm-up to the field or court. Think of your warm-up as a way to prepare your cardiovascular, neuromuscular, and muscular systems in an integrated manner. At the end of a warm-up, you should "have a little lather on you" (i.e., be sweating a little) and your heart rate should be elevated to a state of readiness.

We refer to our dynamic warm-up as dyno, and it includes a series of relaxed skips, rhythmic skips, and dynamic stretches. A good warm-up doesn't rely on a set timetable. Intuitive athletes will feel when their body is ready to play. A tailored warm-up starts with the basic

Skips Within the Dynamic Warm-up Sequence

Why do we skip as opposed to bike, jog, or swim? Skipping taps into the nervous system and an athlete's reactivity and elasticity with the ground, and getting an athlete to be more reactive and elastic will help to make them a better athlete. Skipping is the brain telling the feet what to do. What is between the brain and the feet? The body! If an athlete can get her nervous system to go from opposite ends successfully, then she can get the nervous system to communicate successfully with the rest of her body. Skipping not only taps into the nervous system the way we want, but it also gets the body warm and ready for other activities similar to any other warm-up activity. The biggest advantage is that not only is the body getting ready but the nervous system is as well.

patterns described later in this chapter. It starts with broad-based movements and then becomes more specific. For example, a baseball player will start the warm-up with skips and then progress to movements that mimic the specific stressors they will face during the game. Our position players in baseball follow their warm-up with 50-yard (46 m) buildups. That's a light jog slowly building up to 80 percent to 90 percent of a sprint. During this process, we stress that the athlete try to feel the rhythm of the feet hitting the ground so they can feel the different phases of acceleration. I like to use the example of a car's transmission. Start your run in first gear and slowly build up to sixth. As the run builds up, the feet become more reactive to the ground. The athlete feels the transitions, and by doing this, they are mentally and physically prepping for the day. I like to see the athlete do five to eight buildups. Of course, because we used baseball as an example, the runner starts from a baseball stance just as if they were taking a lead off first. Because a lateral start is unique to baseball, you want to emphasize that in a warm-up.

The complete dynamic warm-up that follows will prepare the body for movement and unique stressor-like lateral starts. Complete each part of dyno for about 10 yards (9 m) in one direction and 10 yards back. If you don't have the tools necessary to measure 10 yards exactly, take 10 giant steps and mark where you end on your 10th step; this equals about 10 yards.

Relaxed Skips

As you complete the skips that follow, keep your upper body loose.

BUTTERFLY SKIP

The first skip in dyno is the simplest and is designed to get the body moving while feeling the ground beneath your feet.

TECHNIQUE

1. Start with a light forward skip (bring one knee up as you hop forward on the other foot, then switch) while swinging your arms back and forth across your body *(a)*.
2. Think about reaching your shoulders with your opposite hands as you swing your arms *(b)*.

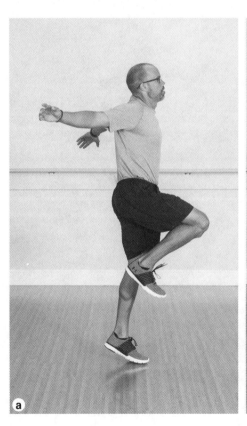
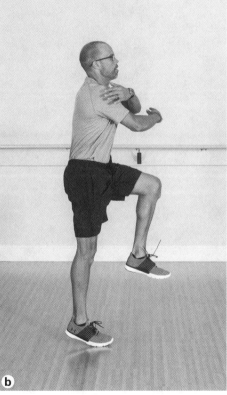

BOTH-ARMS-UP SKIP

This skip uses the same rhythm as the butterfly skip, but the arms swing up and down instead of across the body.

TECHNIQUE

1. Raise both arms and one leg simultaneously.
2. Think about brushing your ears with your biceps on your way up *(a)* and reaching behind your backside on the way down *(b)*.

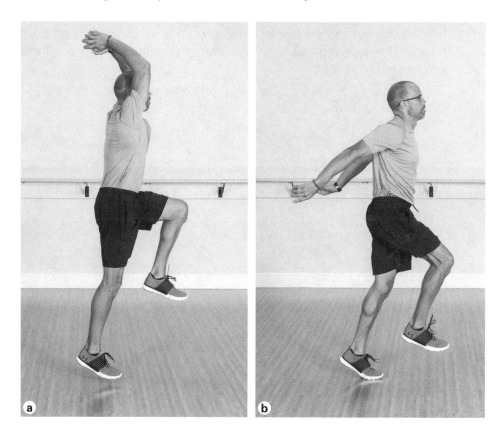

OPPOSITE-ARM, OPPOSITE-LEG SKIP

The last relaxed skip introduces a bit of dissociation for the nervous system. We are separating movement patterns from the upper-and lower-half of the body as well as from right to left. Just like when you're walking, the opposite arm swings every time you take a step. Essentially, this is communication between the right and left side of the brain, but when we are using these movement patterns, we are looking for an over exaggeration of the natural patterns that occur.

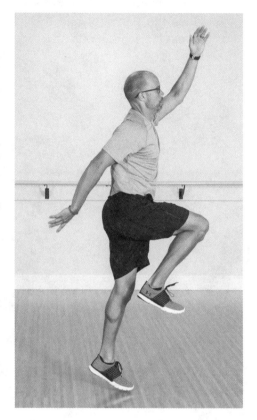

TECHNIQUE

1. Swing your arms up and down, as you did with the both-arms-up skip.
2. Instead of raising the same arm and leg, swing the left arm as your right knee comes up and vice versa.

Rhythm Skips

To find the rhythm of these skips, take a couple of small hops before each skip to find the pattern of ground contact before engaging your arm movements. These skips are the same as above; however, the jumping jack and rhythm skips are now focused on the rhythm or pop effect instead of just the relaxed warm-up skips.

JUMPING JACK SKIP

In this skip, think about popping off the ground through your foot while establishing a rhythm during the skip.

TECHNIQUE

1. Bring your knee to your chest and clap both hands under the knee *(a)*.

2. As the first knee comes down, swing your arms out to the sides, much like a traditional jumping jack *(b)*.

3. Once the first foot hits the ground, pop up with the other foot and repeat the same modified jumping jack motion, clapping under the raised knee *(c)*.

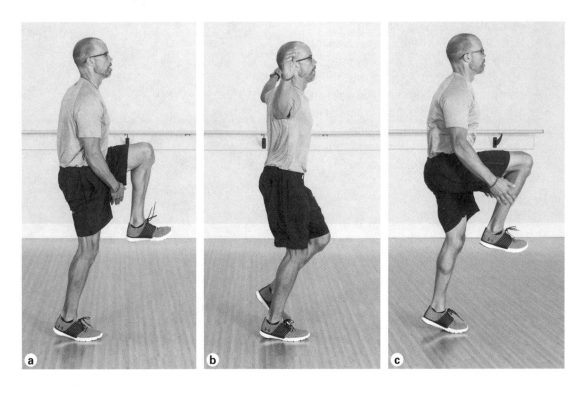

WIDE SKIP

This skip brings your knees out to create nonlinear flexion of the hip.

TECHNIQUE

1. As you skip forward, bring your knee up and out to about a 45-degree angle from your body before returning the foot the ground.

2. Keep your upper body loose by swinging the arms opposite the legs like you would if you were running or jogging *(a, b, and c)*.

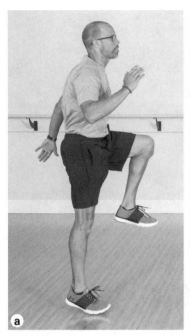
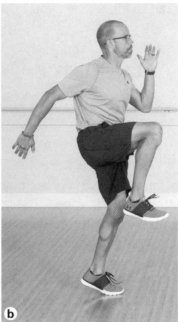
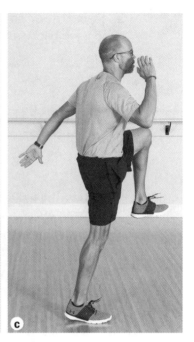

BACKWARD SKIP WITH ROTATION

This is the same as the wide skip, but it is done moving backward.

TECHNIQUE

1. As you skip backward, bring the knee up *(a)* and rotate the hip out (abduct) *(b and c)* through the full range of motion to ensure complete mobility.

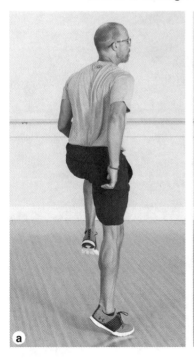
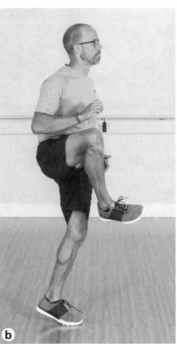
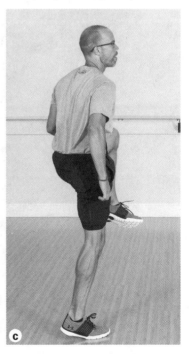

2. Swing the arms opposite the legs like you would if you were running or jogging backward.

LATERAL SKIP

This skip may be the trickiest of the dyno routine, but once the correct rhythm is found, it becomes easier.

TECHNIQUE

1. Turn to the side so you can move laterally. March in place while swinging your arms.
2. Once you have the marching rhythm down, drive the feet into the ground as you move to the side *(a and b)*.
3. The key to this skip is to imagine a stick between your legs that will keep distance between them. This will help you maintain separation so you don't cross over with the back leg. To go left, push off from the left foot. To go right, push off from the right foot.

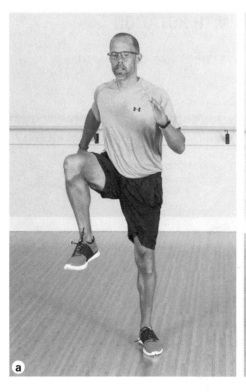 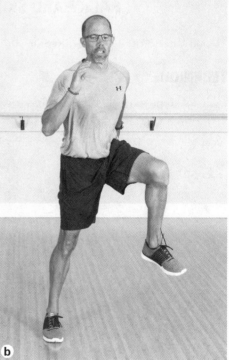

LATERAL SKIP WITH ROTATION

Use the same marching rhythm of the lateral skip and add a crossover.

TECHNIQUE

1. As you perform the lateral skip, cross the back leg in front of the front leg by rotating the back hip up and forward *(a and b)*.
2. Rotate only the back leg forward. Do not rotate the forward leg backward. When going to the right, only cross over your left leg and come back to center each time and vice versa.

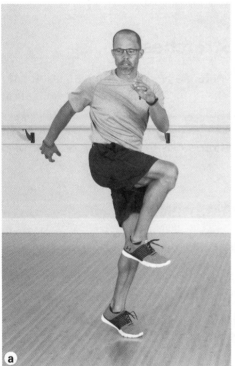
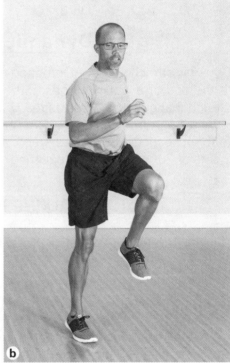

Coaching Tip

We can't express enough how important it is for an athlete to understand movement, and this education starts with skipping. Skipping teaches an athlete not only how to warm up correctly, but also how to move correctly.

The rhythm skips are elasticity exercises that teach an athlete how to become more reactive to the ground. This is important in developing speed, which is essential in all sports. The key factor in reaching full velocity is very little ground-contact time. In other words, the athlete's feet must be reactive and quickly push off the ground. This dynamic skipping series focuses on the athlete's reactivity to the ground. Skipping develops the first aspect of the agility pillar: establishing simple patterns for efficiently responding to the ground.

Dynamic Stretches

Dynamic stretches are not intended to increase flexibility such as stretching at the end of a workout does; rather, dynamic stretches are an activation stretch that gets the muscles ready to go.

When performing stretches that require holding the position, hold for two to three seconds, take three steps, and repeat with the other leg. Perform 2 sets of 20 repetitions on each leg.

WALKING HAMSTRING

The athlete moves forward to limit the time the stretch is held so it does not become a static stretch.

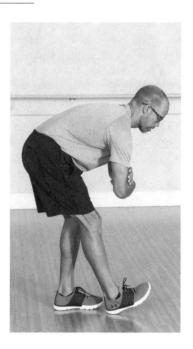

TECHNIQUE

1. Straighten one leg in front of you, point the toes up, and place the heel into the ground.
2. Bend the back leg slightly to allow a deeper stretch.
3. Reach down to either the back of your knee, your calf, or your toes and hold. You can also cross your arms and reach downward with your elbows.
4. Rise with control, take a couple of steps forward, and proceed with the other foot for 10 yards back and forth.

BUTT KICK

The focus of this exercise is to bring the heels back toward your glutes rather than lifting the knees toward your chest. This exercise opens your hips and creates length through the quad.

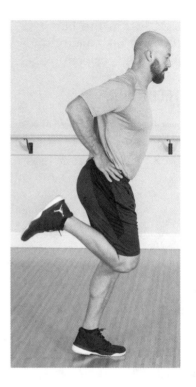

TECHNIQUE

1. Place your hands on your hips and run forward. Keep your hands on your hips to ensure a slight forward lean, mimicking correct running form.

2. As you run, kick your butt with your heels, landing lightly on the toes.

3. Bring the heels up as quickly as possible as you run forward 10 yards (9 m) and back, taking as many steps as possible.

WALKING QUAD

This stretch focuses on loosening the quadriceps by pulling the heel to the backside.

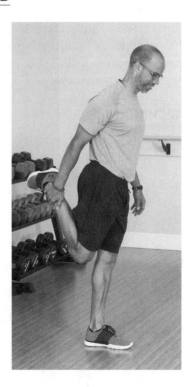

TECHNIQUE

1. Balance on one leg as you raise your foot off the ground behind you.

2. Grabbing the foot or ankle with the hand on the same side of the body, pull the foot toward your backside until you feel a stretch down the front of your leg.

3. To reach a deeper stretch and to activate your hip flexor, lean forward slightly to open the hip a bit more, but don't lean forward too much. This loses the focus of the stretch and you could fall forward.

4. Walk three steps and change legs. Continue for 10 yards (9 m) or a total of 10 stretches.

HIGH-KNEE RUN

Just like in the butt kick, this run focuses on rapidity and taking as many steps as possible.

TECHNIQUE

1. As you run, bring the knees up toward your chest.
2. Think of your legs as rapidly firing pistons moving up and down rather than reaching up and out as in a traditional run.
3. Swing your arms smoothly and strongly to help keep your rhythm. The movement is similar to sprinting.

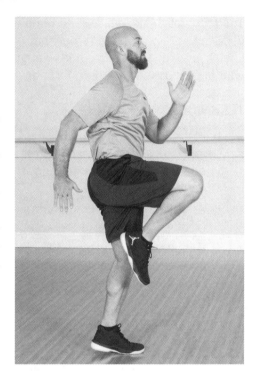

DYNAMIC HAMSTRING

This stretch addresses the higher hamstrings. Although you might not be as flexible, picture yourself as a Rockette in a kick line.

TECHNIQUE

1. Take three steps, kicking up on the third. Take three more steps and kick the other leg. You will take two steps between each kick, alternating the leg that kicks while moving forward.
2. To kick, swing a straight leg as high as you can in front of you without losing your balance. Reach out with your hand to provide a target for your foot.
3. As your leg returns to the start position, stop it as it reaches the ground without letting it swing behind your body.

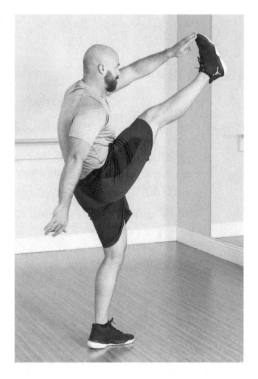

WALKING PIRIFORMIS

The piriformis is a small muscle located behind the gluteus maximus that helps the hip rotate to turn the leg and foot outward. It allows for smooth lateral movement.

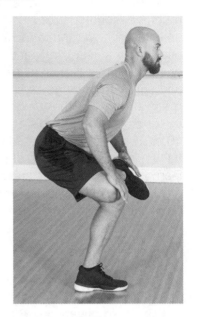

TECHNIQUE

1. As you balance on one leg, bring the other ankle to rest on the knee of the standing leg.
2. Gently apply pressure on your knee with your hand. You should feel this stretch in the outside of your hips as well as your glutes.
3. Take three steps and repeat this on the opposite leg.

TIP

If you want a deeper stretch, bend the knee of the standing leg while pushing down on the top knee. Move your hips back as if you were sitting into a chair behind you.

Once you have completed dyno, you should feel warmed up and neurologically ready for your next series of movements.

Glute Activation Series

Do you know which area of your body is essential for creating speed and power? Your glutes. Because they are involved in most movements, developing speed depends on working them efficiently. Take a look at the best athletes you know and you'll see that they all have a well-developed posterior chain (the muscles along the back of the body). It's no coincidence that they have emphasized this area. They know these muscles are the key to generating speed.

When many young athletes come to us, the first thing their parents say is that they have no clue how to use their lower half. To teach an athlete how to incorporate the lower half in movement patterns depends on their age. For example, it is more difficult to create good patterns in a pitcher who is a high school senior than a younger athlete because of the volume of bad patterns they have repeated over the years. The task is not impossible, it will just take more repetitions from the athlete and a solid understanding of the change that must take place.

We worked with an athlete from a local college who was one of the better pitchers in the state. He came to us his senior year and no matter how much he repeated proper patterns and glute-specific exercises, he was not able to carry over these movements into a game. The lunge or split squat is used often at Beyond Motion. The movement forces an athlete to use their glutes, and this directly carries over to sport in running. When accelerating and sprinting, a lunge or split squat position is shown. Getting the movement stronger in the weight room will make the movement stronger and faster on the field. If this athlete had started training with us when he was 10 to 12 years old, it would be have been a different story. He would not have reinforced a decade of inefficient movements. Instead, he would have learned proper patterns and repeated them easily.

While the gluteal muscles are important for proper movement, they can be overemphasized. In one example, Tiger Woods said he couldn't compete in a tournament because his glutes weren't firing. When your glutes don't fire properly, your movements can become distorted. Think of your glutes as your power zone and shock absorbers. You need them to move effectively because they drive your knees, and your knees drive your ankles and feet. The glutes can be a complex area to train.

The glute activation exercises use a miniband in either a light or medium resistance. You will place the band around both legs, about 3 inches (8 cm) above the knees. Once you have mastered the series with the band above the knees, move the band to about 3 inches above the ankles.

Lateral Movements

Lateral movements stabilize the pelvis and strengthen the medial glute. Think of all of the lateral movement in tennis and pickleball, and how important stability is for volleyball, football, and baseball players.

The following exercises are performed in the same body position. Complete three sets, going about 10 yards or meters down and 10 yards or meters back.

LATERAL GLUTE WALK

This exercise develops the glutes and hip abductors. Maintain the same depth throughout the exercise and the same distance on every step. The imagery we use is to pretend you have a glass of water on each shoulder that you don't want to spill. Use the glutes to take the resistance and keep your upper body quiet.

TECHNIQUE

1. Begin in a squat position with chest lifted *(a)*, and take a large step to the side *(b)*.
2. Bring the other leg in until your feet are about hip-distance apart. Walk laterally for the desired number of repetitions, and then repeat on the other side.
3. Maintain a squared body position so that the shoulders are relaxed and the hips hinge behind your heels.

TIP

Keep the chest lifted and the spine long.

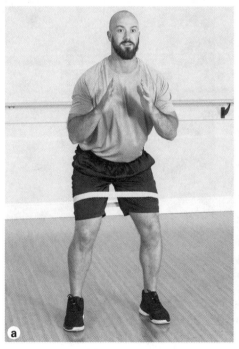
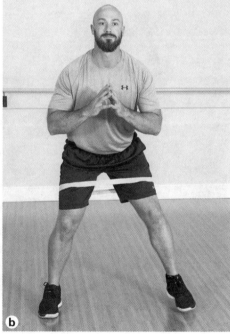

LATERAL GLIDE

This progression creates lateral force. Pushing away is a different action than pushing up like in a jump. The gluteus medius is your lateral mover and your gluteus maximus is your vertical mover.

TECHNIQUE

1. From a squat position, push off the inside of the right foot to bound laterally to the left *(a)*. The feet land a little wider than hip-distance apart.

2. Drag the ball of the right foot until the feet are again hip distance apart *(b)*. Continue for the desired number of repetitions, and then repeat on the other side.

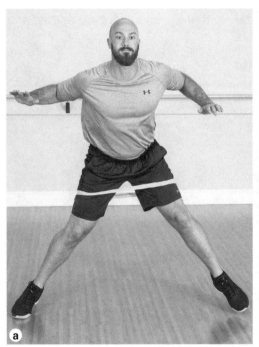 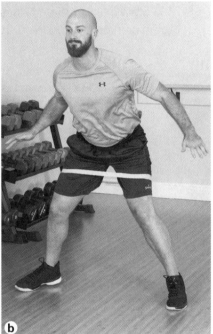

Forward-Facing Movements

This series focuses on your quads, an integral part of the movement chain that starts at the glutes, transfers to the quads, and then to the ankles. Each portion of the chain working together is important for effective movement.

FORWARD 45-DEGREE WALK

Maintain the same depth throughout the exercise and take the same size step each time. Imagine you're in the center of a room and moving forward to a corner. The exercise moves toward the right corner with the right foot and to the left corner with the left foot. To fully engage the glutes, stay low and in control.

TECHNIQUE

1. Start with the feet together in a squat position. Hinge back from the hips, lift the chest, and lengthen the spine.
2. Facing forward, step out 45 degrees *(a)*, and then bring the trail foot forward to meet the front foot. Take the next step with the trailing foot *(b)*. The foot is always moving 45 degrees out (i.e., left foot out at 45 degrees and right foot out at 45 degrees).
3. Keep the body stable and the chest and hips facing forward.
4. Make sure the feet come together between each step.

REPETITION

Continue for the desired number of repetitions, and then turn around and repeat.

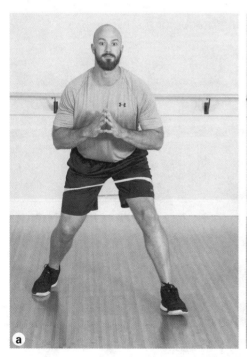
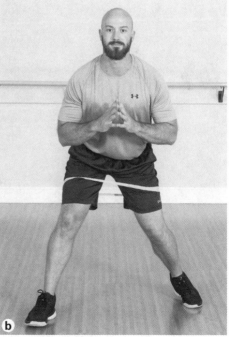

BACKWARD 45-DEGREE WALK

Similar to the forward-facing 45-degree walk, this exercise maintains the same depth and stride length throughout the exercise. The movement is a simple step back and to the side at a wide angle while the upper body remains motionless.

TECHNIQUE

1. Begin in a squat position with the feet together. Lift the chest and lengthen the spine.
2. Take a step backward at a 45-degree angle, maintaining core and back alignment *(a)*. Keep the chest and hips facing forward.
3. Bring the trail leg back to meet the other leg to return to the starting position.
4. Take the next step with the trailing leg in a backward zigzag motion *(b)*.

REPETITION

Complete three sets of 14 steps down and back for 10 yards each way.

VARIATION

Athletes with hip issues can modify the exercise by opening their body toward the foot they stepped back on to allow for rotation of the hips.

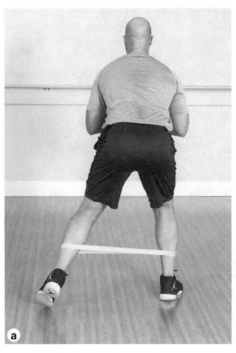 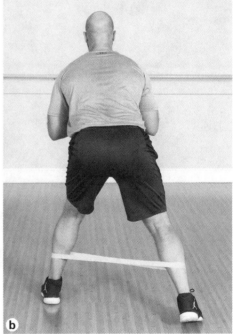

LATERAL TOE TAP

In this exercise, the athlete establishes one leg as a pillar and the other as the mover. Often the standing leg feels like it's getting more work than the moving leg. Lateral toe tap requires balancing as you extend one leg to the side while maintaining a bend in the standing leg.

TECHNIQUE

1. Stand with feet about hip-distance apart, and place the band around both legs about 3 inches (8 cm) above the ankles.
2. Anchor the stationary leg into the ground. The foot is forward and the hips sit back in a slight squat position. The knee is positioned behind the toes, not over them, and directly above the ankle.
3. Lift the working leg to the side and tap the toes on the ground *(a and b)*. Keep the pelvis stable, chest lifted, and spine lengthened.
4. Maintain pelvic alignment so that you do not shift, hike, or twist the hips during the movements.

REPETITION

Tap 20 times on each leg. Complete three or four sets of lateral taps, doing 20 on the left leg, then 20 on the right leg.

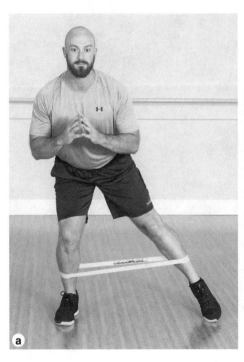
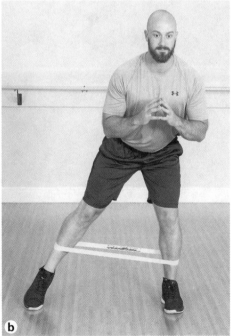

FORWARD TAP

The forward tap is similar to the lateral, but the tap occurs directly in front of you. You may feel like the standing leg is getting more work than the moving leg. Alternate the tapping leg in the same pattern as the previous exercise.

TECHNIQUE

1. Follow the first two instructions for the lateral toe tap.
2. Lift the working leg and tap the foot on the ground in front of you *(a and b)*. Keep the pelvis stable, chest lifted, and spine lengthened.
3. Maintain pelvic alignment so that you do not shift, hike, or twist the hips during the movements.

REPETITION

Tap 20 times on each leg. Complete three or four sets.

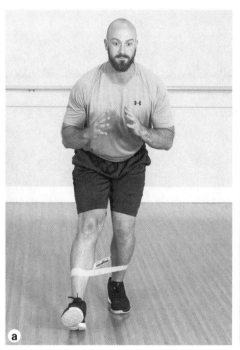
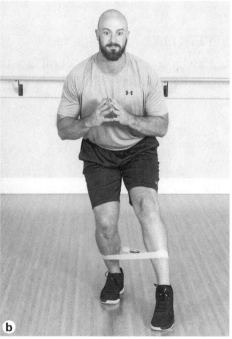

TAP BACK

During this single-leg tap, place the leg directly behind the hips. The glutes and hamstrings should work together to create the movement.

TECHNIQUE

1. Follow the first two instructions for the lateral toe tap.
2. Lift the working leg and tap the foot behind you *(a and b)*. Keep the pelvis stable, chest lifted, and spine lengthened.
3. Maintain pelvic alignment so that you do not shift, hike, or twist the hips during the movements.

REPETITION

Tap 20 times on each leg. Complete three or four sets.

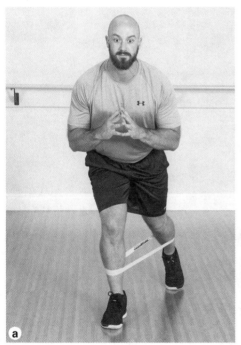
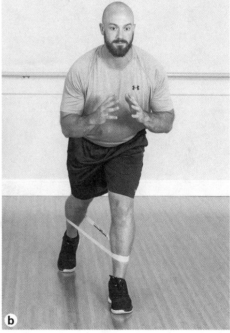

Next Steps

With dyno and glute activation out of the way, you're already more prepared than 99 percent of the athletes out there for anything and everything. These two series create an effective activation workout that can be done on a recovery day or on what I like to call a body-specific day. This is the day to focus on the small stabilizing muscles that enable efficient movement. The next chapter builds on the warm-up you've just learned by focusing on Pilates, which will not only challenge your body, but also your mind. Our most mature professionals who understand performance love Pilates. They feel the instant feedback that no other modality offers. Also, our clients who come to us from the Pilates side and then transitions into weight training have beautiful technique. The mobility and flexibility they have developed through Pilates are attributes essential for all sports and are evident from day one.

PART II | CONDITIONING EXERCISES

5 | Pilates Exercises

Now that you have an idea of how to increase your body awareness, breath control, flexibility, and glute activation, it's time to learn more about Pilates. Pilates is an essential part of a training program that can help you gain a competitive edge.

During Pilates, you work through dynamic flexibility exercises while maintaining your core stability. Professional and elite athletes notice significant improvement in their ability to maintain stability in one section of the body while moving another and to enhance their overall power and performance. This helps them build the muscle relationships needed to gain core strength and flexibility simultaneously and leads to an increase in overall strength, speed, and endurance. Improving core strength while also increasing back flexibility and hamstring length creates a longer stride, which directly increases your speed and agility. This is especially noticeable in track, football, and basketball athletes.

Using the dynamic warm-up techniques in chapter 4 along with the following Pilates exercises will allow you to create unique programs you can use on both your training and recovery days.

Pilates Principles

"With body, mind, and spirit functioning perfectly as a coordinated whole, what else could reasonably be expected other than an active, alert, disciplined person."
—*Joseph H. Pilates*

In chapter 1, we briefly mentioned the six Pilates principles. These are not only fundamental to the method, but they also define it. The six principles are breath, centering, concentration, coordination, flow, and precision.

Think of the six principles as your guidebook. They will tie together the theory, practice, and philosophy of Pilates and be evident in every exercise. By following these principles, you will achieve the true aim of Pilates: a complete body-conditioning program.

Breath

Joseph Pilates says in his book *Return to Life Through Contrology* "Breathing is the first act of life, and the last . . . . Above all, learn how to breathe correctly." Breathing helps to promote natural movement within the body. The breath cycle is a complex process involving both muscles and joints. You will notice the following benefits as your breath control improves:

- Improved circulation
- Removal of toxins from the body
- Stress reduction
- Improved concentration

Centering

The term *centering* in Pilates can be described as finding your center of gravity, or distributing the weight and position of the body so you can move from your center. Centering the body allows you to find and focus on your powerhouse regardless of whether you are standing, sitting, or lying down. Body awareness and centering go hand in hand. Centering allows movement to become more effortless and balanced.

Concentration

In Pilates, concentration is required for performing all movements correctly. The minute you zone out you lose your form and control. Concentration enables quality movement and teaches the mind to be aware of what the body is doing.

Coordination

Think of coordination as the thought process behind the specific movement and the goal of the exercise. By working on coordination, you are working to control your mind and your body so that your movement is fluid and your form is precise.

For example, say a tennis player wants to change their backhand. As they practice this new technique and increase their skill level, the new backhand becomes easier and more familiar. Coordination allows the athlete to become comfortable in the movement and offers direction as they practice this learned skill.

Flow

The word *flow* as applied in Pilates is used just as it sounds. The fluidity of movement joins the exercises so they build on one another. Momentum is never used, but fluidity is. Because you never want to "power through" or bounce while doing a Pilates exercise, control and flow are important. There's a difference between flow and being fluid in your movements and using momentum. Pilates exercises should be completed with control, ease, and fluid, graceful movement. Avoid definite stops and starts for an exercise, which stop the flow of movement.

Flow is necessary for developing movement proficiency. Bridging the movements in a flowing pattern develops a feeling of focus, energy, and proficiency. Pilates is a practice that benefits all activities at every level of fitness. Whether you are a professional athlete or novice mover, you can develop greater strength, endurance, and fluidity in all movements on the field or court by incorporating Pilates into your program.

Precision

Precision is the fine-tuning and execution of each movement for its specific purpose and benefit. The more precisely the movement is performed, the greater the benefit to all movement patterns.

While flow is about creating easy movement, precision is about executing and repeating a correct and exact movement pattern each time. While Pilates movements are fluid, they are also precise. The movements should not be sloppy or haphazard. A "hit point" or particular range of motion is required for each exercise. As you go through the exercises that follow, you will learn the precision required for each movement.

An exercise in Pilates may look similar to another exercise learned in other modalities, but in fact, the precision of the execution combined with the specific breathing patterns for each exercise differentiates it from other exercises. By following the Pilates principles as you perform the exercises in this book, you will gain a new understanding of how your body works and the best tools to help you become an even better athlete.

Your Powerhouse

To fully understand the power of your powerhouse, let's discuss what this term means. Most people think that your core is made up of only the abdominals, specifically the rectus abdominis, or six-pack. However, your core, or powerhouse, is more accurately defined as the center of your body, where you access your power. It incorporates several abdominal muscles, including the rectus abdominis, transversus abdominis, and obliques (see figure 5.1) in addition to the pelvic floor muscles, the muscles surrounding the hip joint, and lower-back muscles, including your erector spinae, and multifidus.

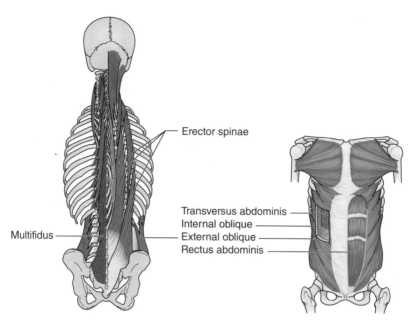

FIGURE 5.1 Posterior view of the multifidus and erector spinae, and frontal view of deep abdominal muscles.

It is believed that Joseph Pilates considered the powerhouse to be the physical center of the body where all Pilates movements should come from. Many Pilates exercises are designed to strengthen the powerhouse and increase strength and flexibility throughout the rest of the body. The goal is of course to keep your powerhouse working consistently throughout each exercise. You should be able to keep your pelvis and spine in the desired position while moving your extremities or your entire body without distorting or compensating during the movements.

When working your powerhouse correctly, your extremities should be able to move in a more fluid manner. People who can't maintain control of this area during a particular movement or exercise often have a weak core and are unstable. They may experience back pain or weakness, tight hips, glutes that won't fire, and poor posture.

A basic understanding of this group of muscles will make it easier for you to know whether you're strengthening the right muscles during your Pilates and conditioning workouts. The powerhouse is, after all, the center of all strength and energy, and you should feel each muscle working hard during every session.

Amy's Coaching Tips

For the past five years, we have had the opportunity to work with Amy, an All-World Gold Ironman triathlete. From her initial evaluation, we knew that she would need to incorporate Pilates into her conditioning program to increase her overall strength and improve her flexibility. While she was a very successful triathlete, we knew she was capable of much more.

"Pilates helped me become a stronger athlete. Having a stronger core and active glute muscles benefit me in all three sports: swim, bike, and run. Swimming with a tight core reduces drag by not zigzagging though the water. And learning how to engage my lat muscles correctly has made me a faster swimmer. On the bike, in the aero bars, a stronger core helps me maintain an aero position. My run has benefited the most. I am able to maintain proper running posture, breathe better, and keep correct running form. The biggest benefit is that I have remained healthy, a.k.a. injury free, therefore, able to train consistently. Consistent training leads to consistent race results.

Out of all the Pilates mat exercises I do, my favorite mat exercise is the roll-up. It took me a long time to learn how to do it properly and I had to work at it. I now have a more flexible spine and better posture, and I am stronger throughout all those little stabilizer muscles. Pilates taught me that I had to learn how to use muscles I didn't know I had."

Amy Rappaport

Pilates Mat Exercises

The foundation for the Pilates mat exercises is formed from Joseph Pilates' original contrology methods. Contrology focused on developing the ability to control the body with the mind. By becoming aware of how your body performs throughout each movement, you will be able to identify your weaknesses and learn new patterns that will help you increase your strength, endurance, and flexibility simultaneously.

For the following exercises, you will need a Pilates or fitness mat and perhaps a small towel. You can use a yoga mat, but a mat that is slightly padded is beneficial for your spine. Although a large repertoire of Pilates mat work is available, the following exercises are the most common and the ones we use with athletes of all ages. From high school to our professional athletes, we include Pilates mat work in their programs.

Warm-Up Exercises

Face it, most of us have tight muscles. Maybe your hamstrings are your sticking point, or your quads and hip flexors give you trouble, or perhaps your back feels tied up in knots. Regardless of where you're feeling a bit stuck, know that you're not alone. Because every Pilates exercise has a work component and a stretch component, it is not necessary to stretch before doing your Pilates workout. And because many of us have tight muscles, the following exercises will prepare your body for the additional workout ahead.

SPINE STRETCH FORWARD

This spine stretch is great for your back and the hamstrings, but more importantly, it is a deep abdominal exercise and prepares the body for additional Pilates exercises.

TECHNIQUE

1. Sit tall, with the crown of your head toward the ceiling. Imagine your shoulders are directly over your sit bones so that you are neither leaning forward nor backward. Shoulders reach wide to the sides and legs are completely extended in front of you with feet flexed slightly wider than your mat. If you have trouble maintaining both a straight spine and extended legs without feeling your spine collapse forward or your quads grip, try sitting on a slightly rolled Pilates mat or blanket folded so it is 2 to 4 inches (5-10 cm) thick. This will open your hips, ease your quads, and lengthen your low back.

2. Inhale and extend your arms in front of you at shoulder height. The palms face down, and your fingers lengthen forward. Keep your arms directly in line with the shoulders, and maintain a fixed width between the arms (a).

3. Exhale as you scoop your belly, tipping your pubic bone toward your nose and your upper thoracic spine into a large C shape. Imagine the shape of a high and tall uppercase C and not a small lowercase c. Don't roll off your sit bones. You should feel as if you are curling, not collapsing (b).

4. From the lowest, deepest point in the exercise, reverse the action and begin to roll up one vertebra at a time. Start to round up through your lower back, then middle back, and then your upper back until the crown of your head is pointing toward the ceiling.

REPETITION
Repeat four times.

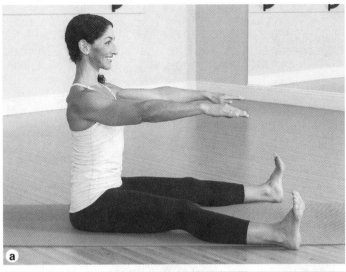

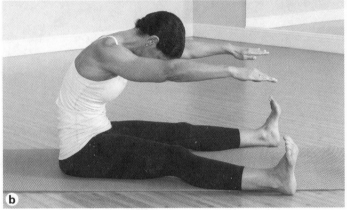

TOE TAP

Toe taps strengthen your powerhouse and lower back, and work on breath control and pelvic stability.

TECHNIQUE

1. Lie supine, with knees bent and feet flat on the mat hip-width apart. Arms are at your sides and pelvis is in a neutral position.
2. Inhale to prepare by bringing the legs into tabletop *(a)*.
3. Exhale, reaching one leg forward from the hip and tapping the toes to the ground *(b)*.
4. Inhale to switch legs and repeat six to eight times.

VARIATION

Begin with a single-leg toe tap four to six times then repeat with the other leg. Once you have mastered that, alternate one tap at a time. Next tap both legs simultaneously. Your range of motion will be shorter than with a single-leg tap.

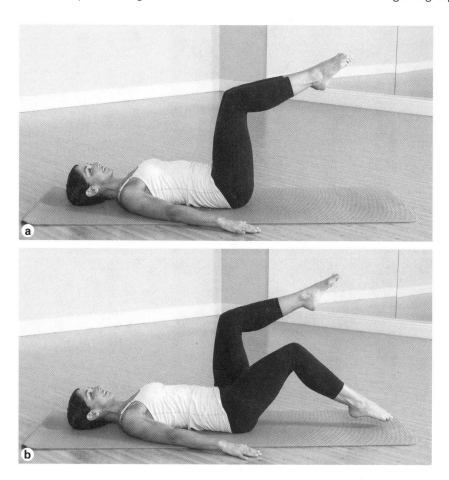

QUADRUPED BIRD DOG

The bird dog is a popular core and spinal stabilization exercise, ideal for reinforcing proper spinal alignment, pelvic stability, and engagement through your entire powerhouse.

TECHNIQUE

1. Come into a quadruped position, making sure that your wrist, elbow, and shoulder are in a straight line on each side and your thumbs are aligned with your armpits. Your hips should be directly over your knees and your ankles in a straight line from your knees. The crown of your head should remain forward throughout (a).

2. Begin by sliding your right leg back, keeping it on the floor until it is completely extended. Once extended, lift it to hip height. Keep your pelvis stable, core engaged, and back long.

3. Raise your opposite arm straight out to shoulder height and level with your ear. Keep your powerhouse engaged and your body in one straight line from head to foot, as if your spine were a string being pulled from the wall in front of you to the wall behind you *(b)*. Sliding your extremities outward before lifting them off the floor makes it easier to keep your powerhouse engaged and pelvis level. The goal is to resist rotating your

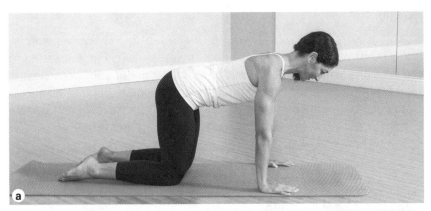

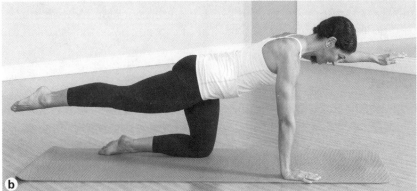

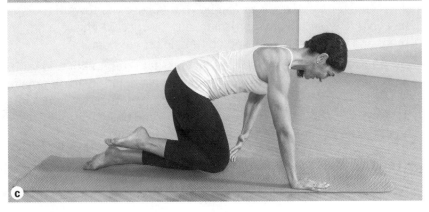

body or allowing the chest or back to sink. If you are unable to remain stable when both your arm and leg are lifted, begin with just the leg movement, then perform only the arm movement, and once you have mastered those, put them together.

REPETITION

Do six to eight repetitions on one side, then switch to the other arm and leg. For a greater challenge, alternate the arm and leg each time for six to eight repetitions on each.

VARIATION

For a basic movement, tap both your arm and leg to the floor as you inhale, and bring them back into a straight line as you exhale. For a more complex movement, bend your knee as it lowers and pull it under your body next to the other knee, keeping it lifted off the floor. Tap the opposite hand to your knee (c). Return to your long position, all while keeping your pelvis level and spine long. Move slowly but fluidly, connecting each movement and breath.

PELVIC CURL

The pelvic curl is ideal for stretching your lumbar spine while learning to engage the muscles of your pelvic floor. It's also great preparation for learning how to create the Pilates abdominal scoop. It is the prep move for articulating your spine into your bridge.

TECHNIQUE

1. Lie supine, with knees bent, feet flat on the mat approximately hip-width apart, and knees and ankles aligned. Look forward toward your knees. Your arms should be alongside your body and shoulders wide and flat on the floor. Your pelvis should be in a neutral position in which you feel as if your coccyx and sit bones were pointing toward the wall in front of you (a).

2. Inhale to prepare. Exhale as you tip your pubic bone toward the sky and feel your low back slightly pressing into the mat (b). This is a tiny movement and your entire back should remain on the floor.

3. As you move, your feet and toes remain flat on the floor and your legs and knees remain still. If you find this challenging, place a small playground ball or folded towel about 2 inches (5 cm) above your knees to activate your adductors and help keep everything in alignment. Maintain a continuous squeeze throughout the movement.

REPETITION

Repeat three to six times.

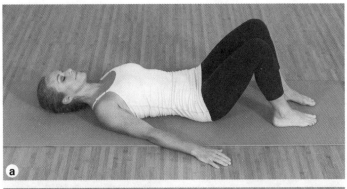

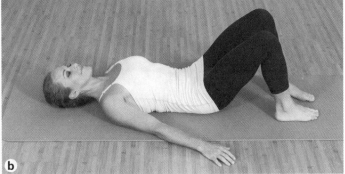

Begin the Work

Now that you have completed the initial stretch, or warm-up, sequence, it is time to begin your actual Pilates workout. Each exercise will not only incorporate all of the Pilates principles you have learned, but also will engage your entire body as opposed to spot training one area at a time.

BRIDGE

The bridge works on articulation of the spine from the base of your tailbone through your shoulder blades. It increases strength in your hamstrings and glutes and connects your breath to your movement.

TECHNIQUE

1. Lie supine, with knees bent and feet flat on the mat approximately hip-width apart. The knees and ankles are aligned. Your arms should be alongside your body and pelvis in a neutral position (a).

2. Inhale to prepare. Exhale, curling the low back into the mat, continuing to lift the tailbone as you peel the spine off the mat one vertebra at a time. Hands and arms continue to press gently into the mat (b).

3. Inhale at the top, then exhale as the body lowers slowly, one vertebra at a time, finishing in neutral position.

REPETITION

Repeat three to six times.

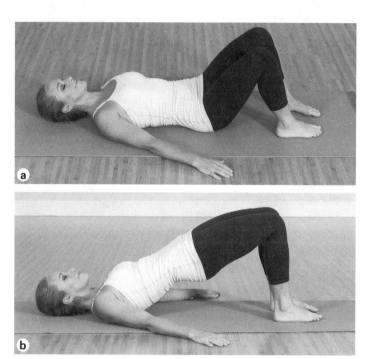

SHOULDER BRIDGE

Shoulder bridge is an intermediate-level exercise. You should master the bridge before trying the shoulder bridge. You must be able to maintain the correct hip and pelvic alignment while performing the leg lift and lower.

TECHNIQUE

1. Lie supine with a **neutral spine**. Your knees are bent and feet on the floor about hip-distance apart and parallel. Extend your arms along your sides, and press the backs of your arms into the mat.
2. Inhale to prepare as you tip your pubic bone toward the sky, creating a scoop through your lower abdominals. Exhale as you press down through your feet and peel your spine off the floor one vertebra at a time until you reach the base of your shoulder blades.

3. Inhale as you bring one knee in toward the chest, then straighten that leg as you reach the foot toward the ceiling while maintaining the alignment of your pelvis and height of your hips *(a)*. The rest of the body stays still. Relax your shoulders and neck; the work is in the abs and hamstrings.

4. Exhale as you lower your leg so that your knees are side by side. As you lower your leg, go for as much length as you can. The knee of your supporting leg, the extended leg, and the tailbone reach for the wall in front of you as the top of your head reaches away in an opposite stretch *(b)*.

5. Repeat three to five leg lifts before lowering your body. Repeat on the other leg.

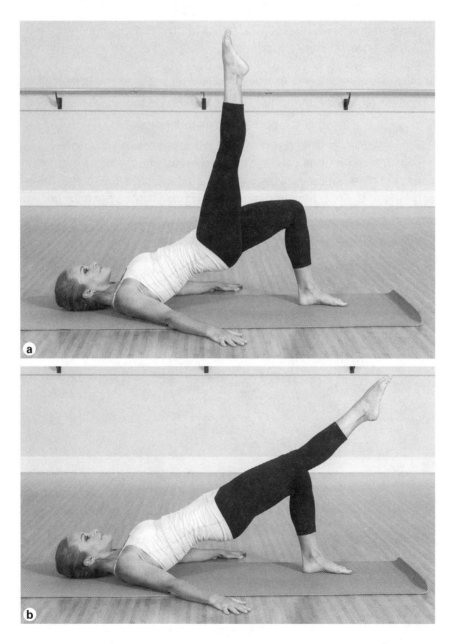

CHEST LIFT

While a chest lift may look like a crunch, it is important to maintain the correct form of the Pilates C-curl throughout the movement. Once you build abdominal strength and understand how to execute this correctly, you will have a solid foundation for many of the supine, forward-flexion Pilates exercises such as hundreds.

TECHNIQUE

1. Lie supine, with knees bent and feet flat on the mat hip-width apart. The palms are stacked at the base of your head, supporting it while the neck and shoulders are relaxed. The pelvis should remain in a neutral position without overtipping or tucking *(a)*.

2. Inhale and bring the chin slightly toward the chest so that your eyes look toward your knees and not the ceiling. There should be enough space under your chin for your fist. Your back should feel long.

3. Engage the internal support system (abdominals).

4. Exhale while contracting the abdominals, allowing the lower spine to sink into the mat as you lift the chest, initiating the movement from the upper spine until the bases of the shoulder blades (scapulae) have risen off the mat. Keep the shoulders drawing down into your back pockets *(b)*.

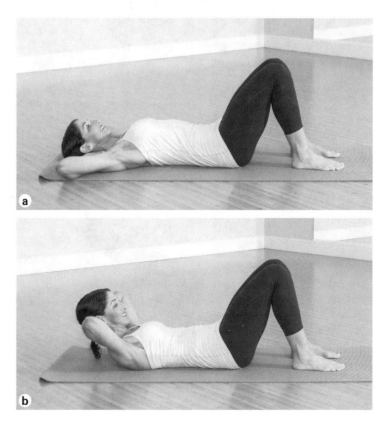

5. Pause and inhale, continuing to draw in the abdominals.

6. Exhale and lower the torso without releasing the abs.

REPETITION

Repeat three to six times.

Series of Five

We refer to the following exercises as the series of five. It includes the hundreds, single-leg stretch, double-leg stretch, crisscross oblique, and hamstring pull. Once you have mastered each exercise independently, try linking them into a flowing movement from one to the next with no break between them.

Each exercise works your entire powerhouse, increases pelvic stability, opens the hip flexors, increases flexibility in the hamstrings, and connects breath to movement.

Rick's Tips

One of the best girls high school basketball teams in our area trains with us. They are an amazing group of athletes with quick hands and great court skills. Being a younger team, they needed to learn how to develop greater core strength, stability, and mobility. They have been working with us on all areas of their performance: strength, speed, and Pilates. One of the biggest changes we have seen is in their Pilates practice. We started the girls with all of the modifications needed to assist them with their tight hips and hamstrings and limited core strength. Within two months, they noticed how much easier the Pilates exercises became. They needed fewer modifications and felt stronger. The following series, known as the series of five, was one of the go-to sessions for these girls.

HUNDREDS

The purpose of the hundreds is to connect your breath to your body, generate heat to warm you up for additional core exercises, and build endurance to enhance overall performance. While the arms pulse to the pace of your breathing, the rest of your body remains still and quiet. The position of your legs can make this a beginner or superadvanced exercise. Trust me, everyone feels the work and is humbled by the challenge of performing it correctly.

TECHNIQUE

1. Lie supine, with the knees bent, feet on the floor hip-width apart, and arms alongside the body *(a)*.

2. Inhale and engage the abdominals.

3. Exhale and roll the upper body into a chest lift, bringing the arms 2 to 3 inches (5-8 cm) from the floor and your palms facing down.

4. Inhale, drawing the abdominals in deeply and begin rhythmic arm presses using a 5 count as you inhale and exhale: Breathe in as the arms pulse above and below the hips for a count of 5, and then exhale as the arms pulse for the next count of 5.

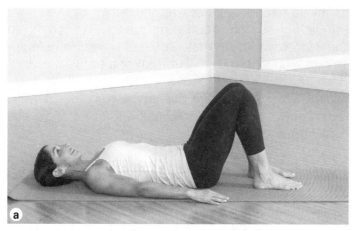

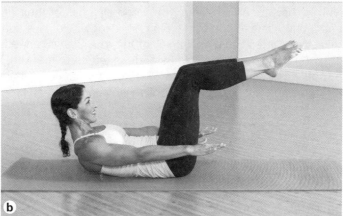

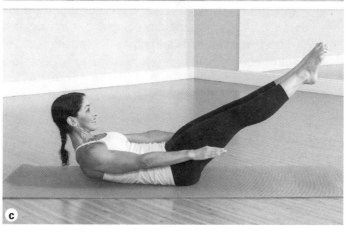

VARIATION

For basic hundreds, keep your feet flat on the floor about hip-distance apart. Once you master this, bring your legs into a tabletop position *(b)*. Once you are able to complete the hundreds easily in tabletop, move to fully extend your legs outward to a 45-degree angle *(c)*.

SINGLE-LEG STRETCH

The single-leg stretch increases the flexibility of your hip flexors, strengthens your core, and stretches your back and legs. Because your upper body remains in flexion throughout the series, your entire powerhouse works, which increases your stamina and endurance.

TECHNIQUE

1. Lie supine. The knees are bent, feet on the floor hip-width apart, and arms alongside the body *(a)*.
2. Exhale while straightening one leg and place the hands firmly on the shin of the opposite leg just below the knee. The knee comes in to the body just beyond tabletop while the other leg extends away fully from the body at a 45-degree angle *(b)*.

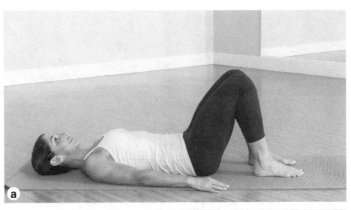

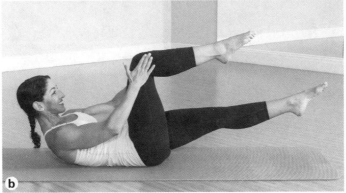

3. Inhale as that leg comes back toward the body, and exhale to extend the other leg while holding the bent leg with both hands.

REPETITION

Repeat, inhaling as the legs pass and exhaling as the single leg extends. Extend each leg 6 to 10 times.

DOUBLE-LEG STRETCH

The double-leg stretch is more challenging than the single-leg stretch. As you inhale, both legs extend toward the wall in front of you and your arms reach straight back to align with your ears. It may be challenging to maintain core control and alignment in this position. On the exhalation, bring the arms and legs back to the starting position.

TECHNIQUE

1. Lie supine, with the chest lifted, and draw the knees toward the chest. The hands rest on the shins, which are parallel to the floor (a).
2. Inhale and reach the legs forward and arms back at a 45-degree angle. Keep the legs together and the arms open, pull the abdominals in deeply, and maintain a neutral spine (b).

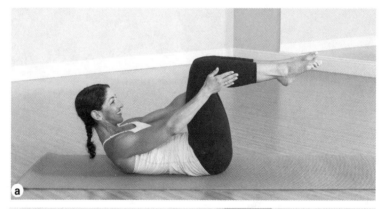

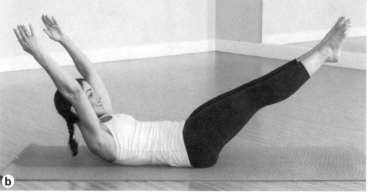

3. Exhale and use the abdominals to bring the legs toward the body and return to the starting position while circling the arms to return the hands to the shins.

REPETITION

Repeat six to eight times.

CRISSCROSS OBLIQUE

Crisscross is the ultimate oblique exercise and, when executed correctly, is challenging. It should feel smooth as you cross from one side to the other without allowing your hips or pelvis to shift or hike. Unlike the old-fashioned bicycle exercise, which many people perform with rapid speed and limited precision, the crisscross is fluid, controlled, and precise.

TECHNIQUE

1. Begin in a supine position, with the upper body in the chest-lift position, legs in tabletop, feet pointed, elbows bent, and head cradled in the hands *(a)*.
2. Exhale and deeply engage the abdominals while straightening one leg and rotating the trunk toward the opposite knee *(b)*.

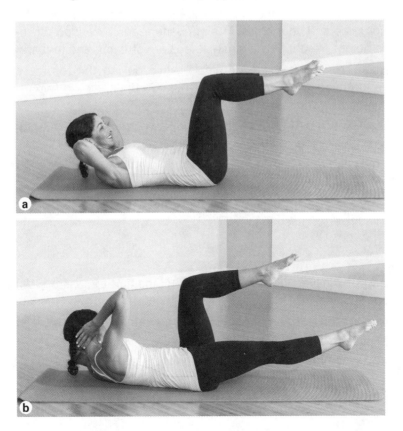

3. Inhale while moving the trunk back to center, bringing the body back to the starting position.
4. Exhale to switch legs, rotating the trunk to the opposite side.

REPETITION

Repeat five times to each side, maintaining a stable pelvis.

TIP

Avoid rocking the body during the movement.

HAMSTRING PULL

The hamstring pull is a favorite for everyone with tight hamstrings. Not only does this provide a challenge for your powerhouse, but because you keep your legs straight throughout the sequence, it is also a great stretch for your hamstrings and hip flexors. As you switch your legs, the lower leg should remain slightly higher than your pelvis so that you feel your transverse abdominals engage rather than your hip flexors and low back.

TECHNIQUE

1. Lie supine, with your upper body in the chest-lift position, one leg lifted toward the ceiling, and hands placed somewhere between the back of your knee and your ankle. The opposite leg is extended off the mat to the height of your pelvic girdle, knees are straight, and feet are pointed.
2. Exhale, engaging the abdominals while pulling the top leg closer to the forehead with two gentle pulses, coordinated with two percussive breaths *(a and b)*.
3. Inhale, keeping the legs straight as you switch legs with control and grasp the opposite leg while lowering the top leg.
4. Exhale and repeat step 2.

REPETITION

Repeat five times on each leg.

TIPS

- Keep your navel pulled in toward the spine and torso lifted to the tip of your shoulder blades.
- Maintain the position of your lower leg when the upper leg is in the pull position.
- Keep your hips stable to avoid rocking.

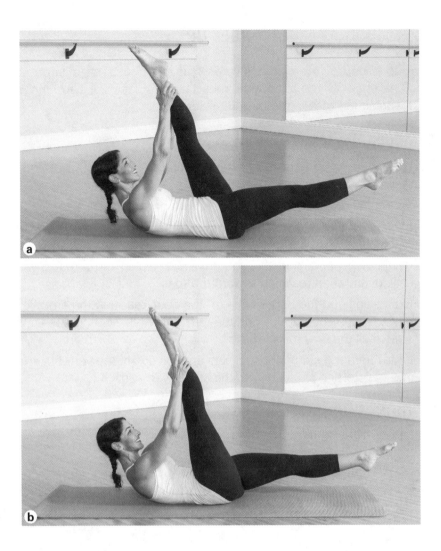

Articulation and Twists

The following exercises create a greater range of motion throughout your spine, increase your core strength, and increase your overall flexibility. Not every person should do every exercise; for example, the roll-up and neck pull can be challenging for some people. Please follow the modifications as needed and remember that in all Pilates exercises, coordinating your breath with your movement is imperative for success. Now that your powerhouse is warm and your spine is a bit looser, it's time to move into additional exercises that increase the challenge.

ROLL-UP

The roll-up is one of the classic Pilates mat exercises. The roll-up provides a great challenge for the abdominal muscles, stretches the hamstrings, and strengthens and stretches the back muscles.

TECHNIQUE

1. Lie supine, with legs fully extended and pressed together and arms reaching overhead *(a)*.
2. Inhale and draw the breath into the back of the ribs.
3. Exhale and draw the ribs down and together, keeping the arms shoulder-width apart.
4. Inhale while engaging the abdominals, bringing the arms toward the ceiling, and then reaching toward the toes.
5. Exhale and curl the upper body off the floor, reaching the arms forward (not using momentum). Continue to roll up while scooping the abs, and stretch all the way forward *(b)*.
6. Inhale to reengage the abs; exhale and roll down one vertebra at a time into the starting position with the arms overhead.

REPETITION

Repeat six to eight times.

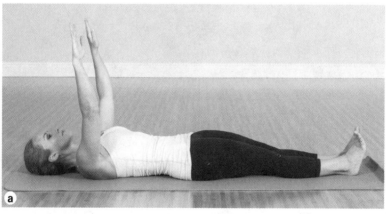

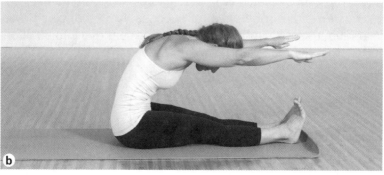

NECK PULL

The neck pull is an intermediate-level Pilates exercise that has little to do with your neck and everything to do with strengthening your powerhouse, stretching your hamstrings, increasing spinal articulation, and strengthening your back muscles. Do the neck pull only after you have mastered the roll-up.

TECHNIQUE

1. Lie in a supine position. Your hands are stacked behind your head, thumbs down the side of your neck, and shoulders relaxed. Exhale to engage your core, bringing your entire back to the floor. Extend your legs, with feet hip-width or touching *(a)*.

2. Take a deep breath in and curl the head and shoulders off the mat. Continue to roll up, exhaling as you draw your abdominal muscles in tight. The hands support your head, but they do not pull on your neck. Your abdominals and pelvic floor engage to do the work of the roll up. Once you have rolled all the way up, continue to roll to create a *C* shape in your spine and arc over your legs *(b)*.

3. Inhale as you return to upright, with your shoulders balanced over your hips. Keep your hands behind or beside your head as you stack your shoulders over your hips and breathe in.

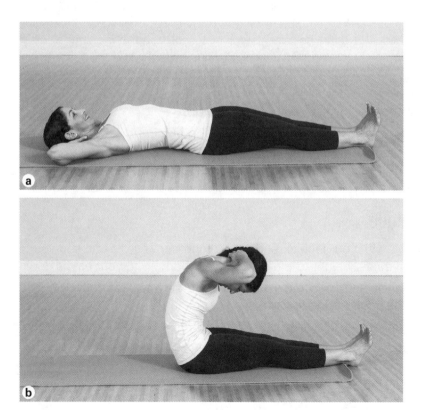

4. To finish one repetition of the move, exhale and roll back down in the same controlled manner in which you rolled up.

REPETITION

Repeat three to six times.

Coaching Tip

If you are a sprinter or a hurdler, it's important that your hips and hamstrings are open enough to maximize your stride length. All other things being equal, the athlete who covers more ground with each stride wins. In addition to helping you win, increased hip mobility can also prevent common pulls and strains that plague sprinters and hurdlers. The tighter your muscles are, the more injuries you may develop.

One of our track athletes is a case in point for the benefit of hip mobility. When she first came to us, her hips, hamstrings, and adductors were super-tight, which caused imbalances in her pelvis and threw off her gait. Her stride length and ability to move over the hurdles was adequate, but we knew she had greater potential. To help her find length in her spine, strengthen her core, and open her hips and hamstrings, we incorporated foam roller work along with a complete repertoire of Pilates exercises. We began with spine stretch, toe tap, chest lift, pelvic curl, and bridge. Next we moved through the series of five and added the spine twist to increase her rotational skills and pelvic stability. It was amazing how quickly her body responded to these movements. As she developed greater stability, we added the side-lying leg series to develop her glute strength. The feedback from this athlete and her coaches was quite positive. Her times decreased, her ability to clear the hurdles with greater ease increased, and she could feel the difference in her body within her first 60 days.

SPINE TWIST

This exercise develops strength in the back extensors and improves spinal rotation through engagement of the abdominals. Keeping your pelvis stable throughout the move trains you to initiate movement from the powerhouse.

TECHNIQUE

1. Sit with your legs extended and together, feet flexed, and your arms at shoulder height to the sides of your body, with your palms down (a).
2. Inhale and engage the abdominals. Exhale and rotate the upper trunk to the right, gazing toward your right hand (b).
3. Inhale as you rotate back to the center, stabilizing the pelvis and abs.
4. Exhale and rotate to the other side.

REPETITION

Repeat three to five times on each side.

TIP

Your legs and feet should remain motionless throughout.

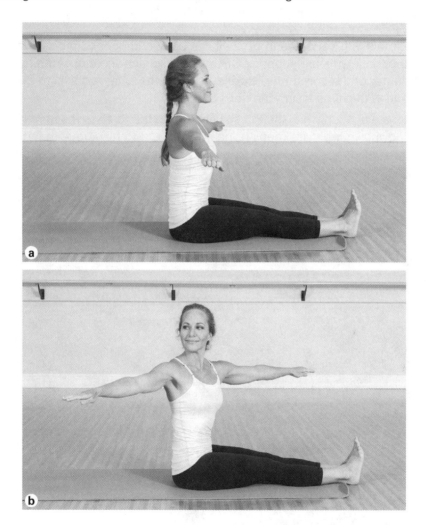

SAW

Saw offers multiple benefits: It lengthens the hamstrings and adductors and develops strength in the back extensors and obliques. Saw is perfect for improving spinal rotation and articulation through engagement of the abdominals.

TECHNIQUE

1. Sit tall with your legs in front of the body and opened a bit wider than the mat. Arms are supported from the midback and elongated from the center of the collarbone, extended out to the sides, parallel to the floor, and with palms facing the floor *(a)*.

2. Inhale to deeply engage the abs and rotate the torso to the right without moving your pelvis, keeping the arms and head moving with the trunk.

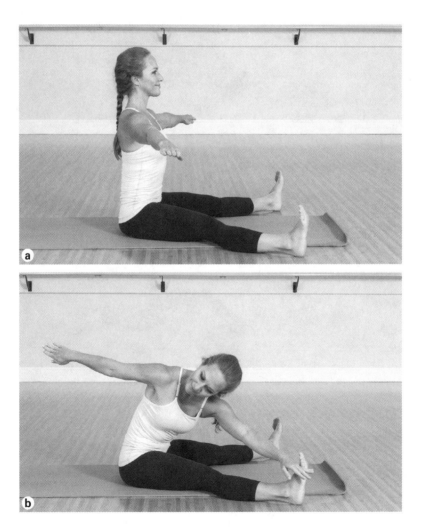

3. As you exhale, direct the left shoulder forward toward the right leg, extending the left arm, and reaching the hand past your toes. Simultaneously, your right arm should be reaching back behind you. While your body rotates on the axis from one side to the other, your arms do not move but remain constant with your torso *(b)*.

4. Inhale and return to center.

REPETITION

Twist and change direction. Repeat three to five times to each side.

Side-kick Series

The side-kick series is ideal for athletes who want to strengthen their glutes, transverse abdominals, and obliques and the group of hip-stabilizing muscles. You know you're doing these correctly when you feel your glutes burn during these small, controlled movements. They should feel controlled, fluid, precise, and relatively small. The side-leg series works the glutes, hips, and thighs. The most important thing to remember while performing these exercises is to stabilize your core.

Among the exercises in this series are the front and back kick, the lift and lower, and circles in both directions, which all start from the following setup position. Begin by lying on your side with your bottom hand under your head and your elbow reaching toward the wall. Your other hand is placed flat on the floor in front of your navel and your elbow reaching away. Your top hand should be far enough away from your chest to prevent your shoulder creeping toward your ear. Your shoulders are relaxed and eyes focused straight ahead so that your neck is in the correct position. For more advanced work, your legs should be stacked on top of each other in a straight line from your pelvic girdle down to the side of your ankle bone. If you need to modify, the legs may be brought to about a 45-degree angle in front of your body.

FRONT AND BACK KICK

Front and back kick increases your range of motion and control as you move your leg slightly in front of and behind your midline while maintaining your entire leg at the height of your hip. As you kick forward, you will feel a contraction of your core as well as a stretch in your hamstrings and glutes. As you kick back, you will feel a sensation of opening your hip flexors while working your core and engaging your hamstring and glutes. This exercise is a front and back kick, so the movement kicks to the front of the body and to the back of the body. Flex the foot while kicking forward, and point the foot while kicking back. The range of motion should be where nothing else in the body moves. The leg movement requires complete stability from the rest of the body.

TECHNIQUE

1. Exhale, flex the foot, and sweep the top leg as far forward as possible without tucking the pelvis (posterior tilt) *(a)*. Keep the pelvis and torso still.
2. Inhale, point the foot, and sweep back as far as possible while elongating the leg and keeping the torso still *(b)*.

REPETITION

Repeat 8 to 10 times on each leg.

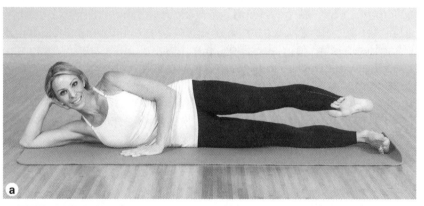

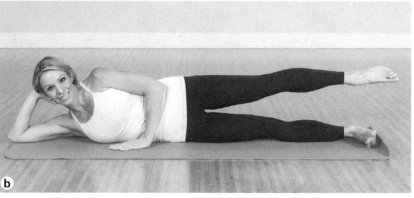

LIFT AND LOWER

The lift and lower works your abductor and adductor muscles while maintaining your core control and alignment.

TECHNIQUE

1. Inhale and engage the underside oblique abdominals, stabilize the bottom leg by pressing your entire leg into the floor *(a)*, and lift the top leg to hip height *(b)*. Your foot remains in a parallel position so that your little toe and heel remain level. Make sure your foot and leg are not rotating.

2. Exhale to lower with control to your starting position.

REPETITION

Repeat 8 to 10 times on each side.

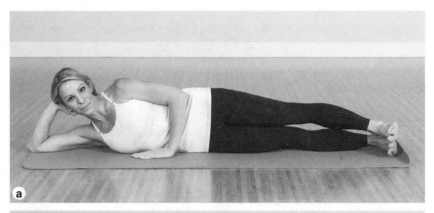

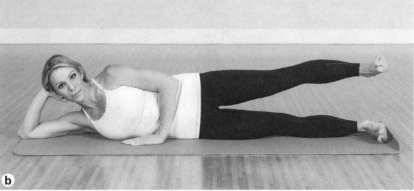

CIRCLE

Circles require control, precision, and flexibility. When you're new to this exercise, the movement should remain small and performed over the lower leg rather than moving in large circles that might create instability throughout the rest of your body. As your strength and flexibility improve, your range of motion may increase; however, this is not required to gain the benefits of this exercise. Regardless of the size of the circle, you will feel your glutes fire as your entire core works to stabilize the rest of your body. Remember the side-kick series is about control, not about how large your range of motion is.

TECHNIQUE

1. Inhale and engage the abdominals, lengthen through both sides of the body, stabilize the bottom leg, and lift the top leg to hip height *(a)*.
2. Exhale and circle the top leg in a forward motion while keeping the hips stable *(b)*.
3. Inhale and continue to bring the leg forward as you complete the circle.

REPETITION

Repeat this motion 8 to 10 times, and then reverse the direction of your circles.

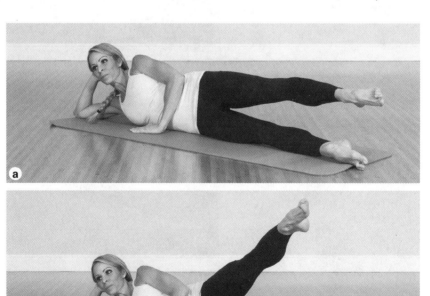

UPPER AND LOWER LIFT

Working control and stability is important for upper and lower lift. Keep your body stable as you work your adductors during this sequence.

TECHNIQUE

1. In the beginner variation, the arm extends to align the head with the spine. The arm position of fully extended under the head is a good option for people with neck or shoulder issues who may have an issue being elevated. It can be used for all of the side-kick series.

2. Inhale and engage the abdominals, stabilize the bottom leg, and bring the top leg to hip height. The ankle, knee and hip should ideally be in a straight line with the pelvic girdle.

3. Exhale and bring the bottom leg to meet the top leg *(a)*.

4. Inhale and lower both legs together *(b)*.

REPETITION

Repeat six to eight times on each side.

TIP

Keep the lifted leg stable; don't lower it to meet the bottom leg. This exercise can be done with the legs in parallel or in external rotation.

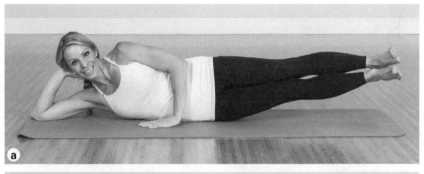

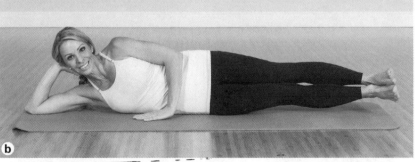

SIDE-LYING CLAM

The side-lying clam exercise strengthens the hip abductors, such as the gluteus medius. It is commonly used in the rehabilitation of lower-back pain and hip injuries. It also teaches pelvic stability and strengthens the glutes.

TECHNIQUE

1. With one hip lying above the other, bend the hips to approximately 45 degrees and bend the knees to 90 degrees. Your feet are in line with your back, as if you were placing them on the back wall.
2. Take a deep breath in and as you exhale, pull your navel to your spine *(a)*.
3. Inhale to prepare, then exhale as you reach your top knee toward the sky while keeping your feet in contact with one another *(b)*.
4. Inhale as you hold; exhale to bring the leg down to the starting position.
5. Focus on maintaining the alignment of the body during the leg movement.

REPETITION

Repeat 5 to 10 times on each leg.

TIP

If done correctly, you should feel the muscles around the back of the hip bone (gluteus medius and minimus) working hard.

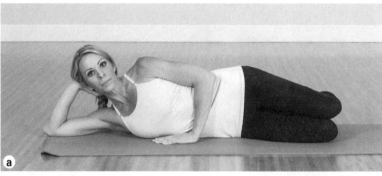

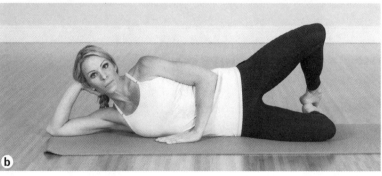

Back Strength and Flexibility

It is important for everyone to work on extension in the thoracic spine (midback), but it is especially important that athletes develop strength and flexibility in this area to counterbalance the forward-facing movements that dominate so many of their activities. Think about a golfer leaning slightly forward over their club, or how basketball players are positioned as they dribble the ball down the court. Swimmers practice thousands of laps over the course of a year, and each stroke uses movements that pull the spine and shoulders slightly forward, typically creating tighter chest and back muscles. By working to open the front of the chest and develop greater strength throughout the back, an athlete can develop better quality movement patterns that are more fluid. The following prone exercises are our go-to exercises for anyone looking to increase strength and flexibility in their middle and upper thoracic area. Many sports create postural imbalances and inconsistent musculature development from one side of the body to the other. In addition to these imbalances, many sports including running, swimming, cycling, tennis, and golf require a more forward posture. Compare it to the posture of a ballet dancer, which is quite tall and lengthened. Exercises that assist in developing greater strength throughout the back extensors and create more openness through the chest will improve not only posture, but also performance.

SWAN

The swan is an extension exercise that opens the front of the body; expands the chest; and stretches the abdominals, hip flexors, and quadriceps. Throughout swan, the abdominals stay engaged while the shoulders, back, inner thighs, pelvic floor, glutes, and hamstrings are at work.

TECHNIQUE

1. Lie prone on the mat. Keep your arms hugged in close to your body as you bend your elbows to place your hands under your shoulders. Shoulders should be away from the ears, and elbows point to the back wall. The legs are typically close together, but it is OK to do this exercise with the legs hip-distance apart.

2. Engage your abdominals by lifting your navel away from the mat. The abdominals remain lifted throughout the exercise. Maintain a connection between the front of the hips and the floor *(a)*.

3. As you inhale, lengthen your spine, sending energy through the top of your head as you press your forearms and hands into the mat to support a long upward arc in the upper body. The elbows are close to the body and should feel as if they brush past your ribs, the head stays in line with the

spine, and the hips stay on the mat. Protect your lower back by sending your tailbone down toward your heels *(b)*.

4. As you exhale, keep your abdominals lifted while lengthening your spine as your torso sequentially returns to the mat: low belly, mid belly, low ribs, and chest.

REPETITION

Repeat swan three to five times using an even, flowing breath to support the movement.

VARIATION

If you find it easier to exhale into extension, you can; just make sure to find length throughout the front and back of the body so that you don't compress your lumbar spine.

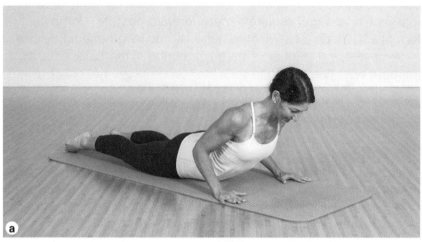

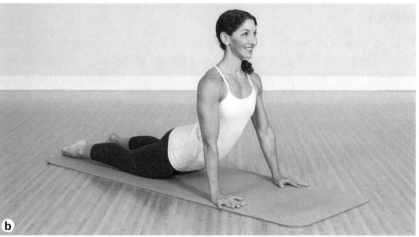

SWIMMING

Swimming strengthens your back, hamstrings, and glute muscles and improves your posture, mobility, and stability. This exercise challenges the core and engages the deep abdominal muscles, helping you improve body alignment.

TECHNIQUE

1. Lie prone with your arms extended in front of the body, palms down. The knees are straight and feet are slightly pointed (a).
2. Inhale to draw the abdominals in while raising the chest, arms, and legs slightly off the mat.
3. Avoid rocking the body by keeping the pelvis stable and the hip bones pressed into the mat.
4. Exhale and raise one arm and the opposite leg. Inhale and switch sides (b).
5. When finished, inhale with the chest, arms, and legs slightly off the mat, and then exhale to lower slowly.

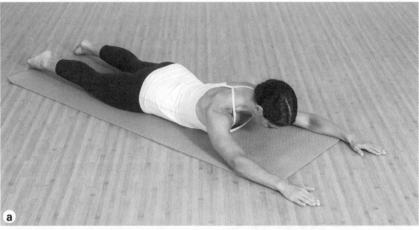

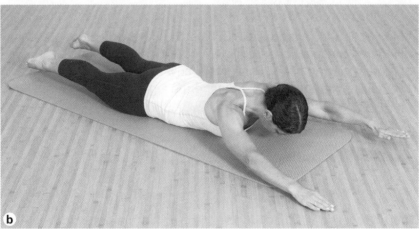

REPETITION

Using this breathing pattern, continue with opposite sides for a count of 10, keeping your hands and feet off the floor throughout.

VARIATION

If you find that it is too challenging to keep your arms and legs off the floor simultaneously while keeping your body still, work one part at a time as follows.

1. Engage the core, keep your legs on the floor, and lift the arms off the floor, swimming with just your upper body.
2. Rest and regroup before working the lower-body swimming action with straight legs. The arms are on the floor, head and neck in a neutral position about 2 inches (5 cm) from the floor, and body still.
3. Once you have mastered the arms and legs separately, perform the exercise with both the arms and legs together.

SINGLE-LEG KICK

The single-leg kick focuses on the hamstrings and glutes. The hamstrings extend the hip and flex the knee in activities such as walking and running. The single-leg kick is also a great way to work your powerhouse and keep your midback engaged. Practice keeping your abdominals lifted, chest open, and shoulders stable while maintaining a long, low back.

TECHNIQUE

1. In prone position, place the hands on the mat, elbows pointing back toward the feet, legs stretched long on the mat, and toes pointed so that the top of the foot presses into the floor *(a)*.
2. Inhale, deeply engage the abdominals, and bend one knee to bring the foot in toward the glute.
3. Flex the foot as it pulses towards the glutes with a brisk 2-count pulse *(b)*.
4. Exhale as the legs switch. Exhale to pulse into the glute, inhale to lengthen the leg. For a beginner version, repeat eight kicks on one leg before changing sides. For a more advanced version, alternate so that you pulse with two pulses. Extend the leg so it's back on the floor and change to the other side.

REPETITION

Repeat a total of 6 sets, which is 12 movements.

TIP

Stay lifted in your shoulder girdle, and engage and lift the abdominals throughout the movement.

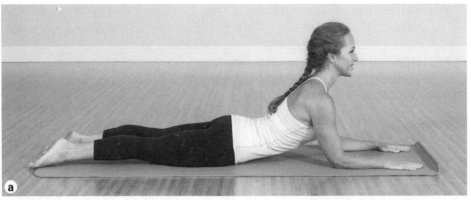

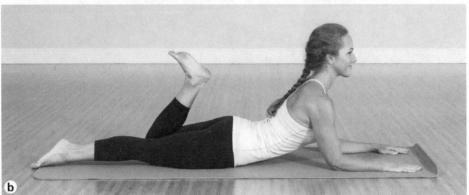

DOUBLE-LEG KICK

The double-leg kick is a powerful back-extension exercise. It targets the back extensors, glutes, and hamstrings and requires support from the entire body.

TECHNIQUE

1. Lying prone, lengthen the legs and place the hands behind the back. The elbows are bent. Rest one cheek on the mat.
2. Inhale and lift both legs a few inches off the mat. The feet are gently pointed.
3. Exhale and bend both knees, bringing the heels toward the glutes in a pulsing manner *(a)*. Pulse two times towards the glutes as you exhale and with an inhale, the legs extend back to straighten. The legs stay together throughout the movement.
4. Inhale and extend the legs while lifting the chest off of the floor and reaching the arms back toward the heels, turning the head to look straight down *(b)*.

5. Exhale while lowering the other cheek to the mat, bending the arms and bending both knees to bring the heels toward the glutes in a pulse.

REPETITION

Repeat six times on each side.

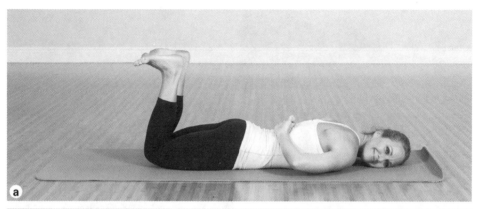

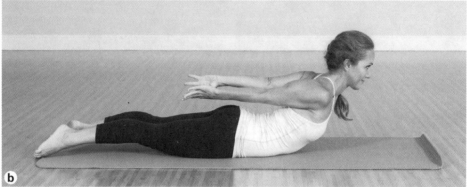

Rolling, Articulation, and Balance

Rolling exercises rely on fluid movement, body and breath control, and, of course, the ability to roll on your spine. They can be great additions for anyone who needs to stretch their spinal extensors and maintain control of their core; however, they should not be performed by people with cervical spine issues.

ROLLING LIKE A BALL

This exercise stimulates the spine, deeply works the abdominals, and connects the flow of movement and breath in the body.

TECHNIQUE

1. In a tall, seated position, round the upper body, bend the knees, and lift the feet off the floor. Wrap the arms around the legs with the palms on the shins *(a)*.

2. Inhale, deeply engaging the abs, and roll onto your back, keeping the head off the floor and maintaining the *C*-curve in the spine *(b)*. Keep your rolled position throughout the exercise.

3. Exhale to roll up to find your balance in the seated position. Use your breath to keep this exercise controlled and flowing.

REPETITION

Repeat six to eight times.

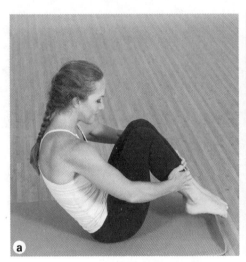
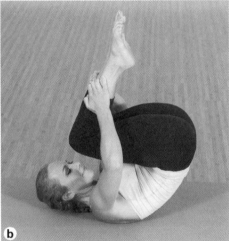

OPEN-LEG ROCKER

Open-leg rocker is a great abdominal workout, using both core stabilization and spinal articulation while requiring balance and control. You will have to use sequential control between the upper and lower abdominals, and keep your abdominals engaged in a deep scoop. Continuous breathing is required to keep this rolling exercise flowing and controlled. Note: If you have back or neck problems or tight hamstrings, use this exercise as a balance exercise without the rolling.

TECHNIQUE

1. Sit in a balanced position with the legs extending toward the sky, shoulder-width apart. Hold your ankles with your hands, if flexibility allows, and straighten the legs fully while you maintain a straight back *(a)*.

2. Inhale, deeply engaging the abs and rounding the back, initiating the movement from the low spine, and rolling back to the shoulders. Keep your head from touching the mat *(b)*.

3. Exhale and roll back up, keeping the spine rounded and then extending it when returning to the starting position. Balance for a moment.

REPETITION

Repeat six to eight times.

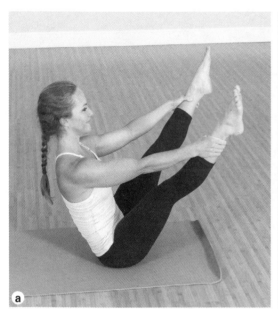
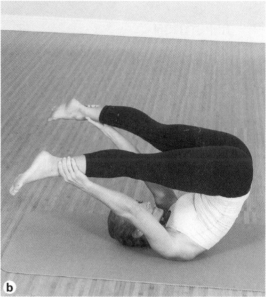

LEG PULL

Leg pull is a core strength builder that engages every part of your body. By lifting one leg off the floor, you introduce instability that challenges your abdominals and shoulders and opens the muscles of your chest.

TECHNIQUE

1. Begin by sitting with your legs straight out in front of you, your core deeply engaged, your back as straight as possible.

2. Place your arms on the mat under the shoulders, palms down, fingers rotated slightly out toward the side. Lift the hips off the mat with the legs extended and toes pointed. Work to press your entire foot into the floor without allowing it to lift or roll *(a)*.

3. Inhale while engaging the abdominals, maintaining the support of the body.

4. Exhale and lift one leg off of the mat *(b)*.
5. Inhale and lower the leg back to the mat.
6. Exhale and lift the other leg off of the mat
7. Inhale and lower the leg back to the mat.

REPETITION

Repeat three to five times on each side.

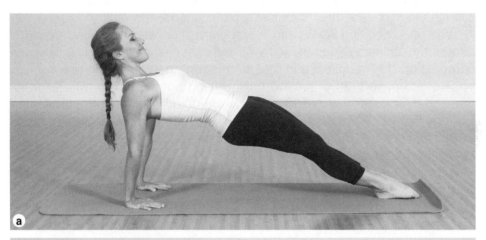

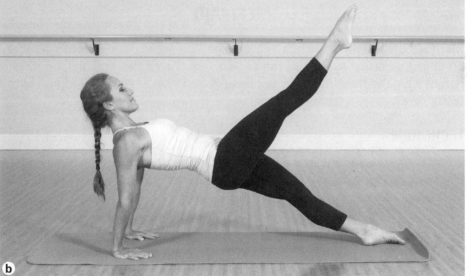

One-Sided Sports

Living in Florida, we work with a large number of tennis and pickleball play-ers. The fitness demands on these athletes are high. Tennis and pickleball require agility, flexibility, balance, range of motion, power, timing, and endurance. If your core muscles are weak, your body will become slower and tire more quickly, forcing other muscles to overcompensate while reducing your effectiveness.

Many sports are considered one sided. This means that sports such as lacrosse, tennis, golf, pickleball, baseball, and softball are typically played with one side of the body. Most people are not ambidextrous, so they hit or swing with the same side over and over instead of hitting with one side and the next with the other. As a result, many players have muscular imbalances between their dominant and nondominant sides. These imbalances can lead to injuries in their shoulders, back, knees, and hips.

When incorporating Pilates into the program of athletes who play one-sided sports, the athletes experienced five significant changes during training and competition: 1.) An increase in their core strength improved stroke control, power, and speed. 2.) Improved balance and control led to quicker reaction and directional changes. 3.) Improvement in muscle control prevented overuse injuries. 4.) Increased flexibility in the back and hamstrings reduced overall injuries. 5.) Improved body awareness and concentration improved overall performance.

We incorporate the next group of exercises with these athletes to counterbalance the work they do on the court and field. The sequence strengthens and opens the muscles they rely on.

MERMAID

Mermaid unilaterally stretches and engages the intercostal muscles (primary breathing muscles) as well as the back extensor muscles and quadratus lumborum (QL). The powerhouse must be engaged to maintain the integrity of the torso.

TECHNIQUE

1. Sit with your legs in a Z-sit or cross-legged position. Inhale to prepare, and imagine lengthening your spine toward the ceiling. Exhale to draw your navel to your spine *(a)*.

2. Start with the arm on the side opposite the front leg. As you inhale, raise it overhead and reach up and over, keeping the arm in alignment with your ear, shoulders relaxed, and the head toward the back wall *(b)*. Don't allow your head and neck to pull forward or drop.

3. The hand closest to your back knee can pull back on this knee to increase the stretch in your QL as long as you maintain both of your hips squared to the front and your glutes firmly planted on the mat.

4. With the extended arm, think of reaching toward the point where the wall and the ceiling meet. This will help you keep the spine long and avoid excessive disc compression.

5. Exhale to return to the starting position.

REPETITION

Repeat three to five times, then change leg position and perform the exercise with the other arm extending.

TIP

If you choose the cross-legged position, the arm on the same side as the front leg stays to your side on the floor. When you change sides, cross the other leg in front. The rest of the exercise remains the same.

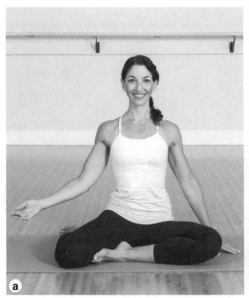
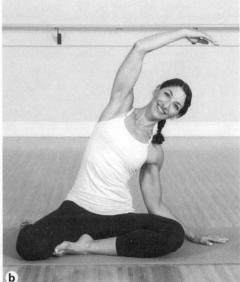

ROLLOVER

Rollover focuses on control. It will stretch your back and hamstrings and make your abdominal muscles work like crazy. Don't allow your legs to flop over your head to the floor, and make sure your body is warmed up properly before you do the rollover. This is a more advanced exercise, and if you have back or neck issues, it might not be right for you.

TECHNIQUE

1. Lie supine, with your arms along your sides and palms down. Your neck is long with lots of space between your shoulders and ears, and your chest is open and eyes forward, looking at where the ceiling and wall meet.

2. Knees are bent and feet are flat on the floor *(a)*. Bring your legs to a tabletop position and then extend them straight up toward the ceiling so that your legs and torso create a 90-degree angle. Keep your tailbone on the floor *(b)*.

3. Inhale to prepare, and exhale as you bring the pelvis off the floor and reach the legs overhead, working to touch your toes to the floor.

4. Inhale to pause at the top while maintaining a round spine as the feet reach to the floor. Spread the legs about shoulder-width apart and flex the feet *(c)*.

5. Exhale, slowly rolling the spine back down to the mat, keeping the legs apart and the abdominals engaged and lowering the legs to the starting position *(d)*.

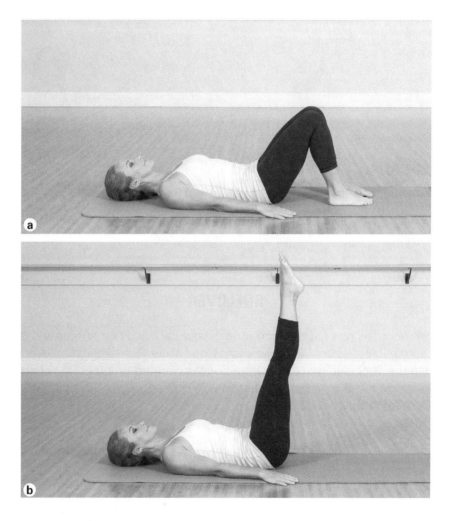

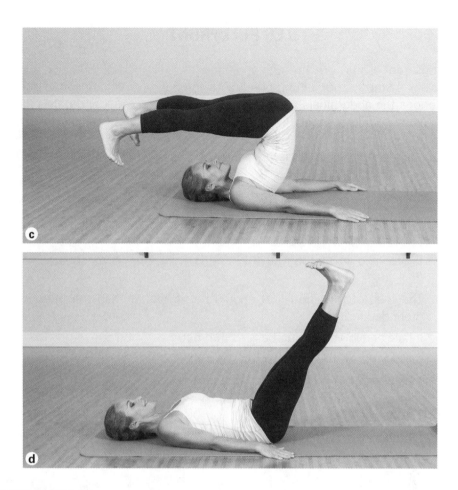

REPETITION

Repeat three to five times and then reverse, beginning with the legs open and closing them while overhead. Perform in that order three to five times.

VARIATION

To simplify this exercise, avoid the actual rollover and perform a lift and lower.

1. Start with your legs extending toward the ceiling, powerhouse completely engaged, and your entire back in contact with the floor.

2. Exhale to lower your legs to about 45 degrees or to the lowest point where your neck is still long, eyes forward, chest wide, shoulders and back in contact with the mat, and core deeply engaged.

3. Inhale to bring the legs back to the 90-degree angle, feet toward the ceiling.

4. This variation provides a core challenge and is safer for people with back and neck issues.

LEG PULL FRONT

Leg pull front builds core strength and engages every part of the body. It takes the plank a step further. Lifting one leg off the floor introduces instability that challenges the abdominals and shoulders to keep the trunk and pelvis stable as you move. While it engages many muscles, you will first feel it in the calves, which is the primary target. Secondary muscles engaged are the hamstrings, glutes, quadriceps, groin, abdominals, and shoulders.

TECHNIQUE

1. Begin in a plank position, hands directly under the shoulders.
2. Inhale to engage the abdominals, and maintain the support of the body *(a)*.
3. Exhale and lift one leg off the mat, keeping the pelvis squared to the floor *(b)*.
4. The toes of the lifted foot should be no higher than the heel of the grounded foot.
5. Inhale and lower the leg back to the mat.
6. Exhale and lift the other leg off the mat.
7. Inhale and lower the leg back to the mat.

REPETITION

Repeat three to five times on each side.

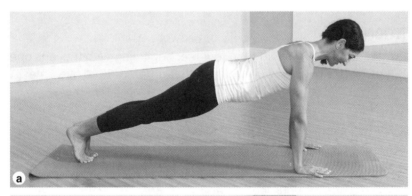

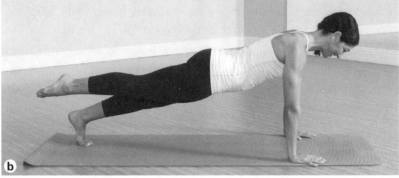

Teaser Series

Teaser is one of the most challenging of the Pilates mat exercises. It strengthens your entire body and incorporates all of the abdominal muscles, spinal extensors, and hip flexors. We start with teaser prep.

The goal for both the teaser prep and the full teaser exercise is to strengthen your back extensors and abdominal muscles, and to perfect articulating the spine into and out from the movement, which prevents the use of momentum or back strain. One thing to remember with both the teaser prep and the full teaser exercise is that your breath will assist getting you getting into and out of the movement correctly. Always inhale to prepare and exhale to move.

TEASER PREP

Teaser prep is a great introductory exercise as opposed to the full teaser, which is quite challenging. Teaser prep is great if you're just beginning your Pilates practice or if you have tight hamstrings, hip flexors, quads or a tight back. You should feel your adductors working as you squeeze your legs together.

TECHNIQUE

1. Lie supine on your mat, legs in tabletop. Inhale as you bring your arms overhead, nod your chin toward your chest and begin to roll your upper

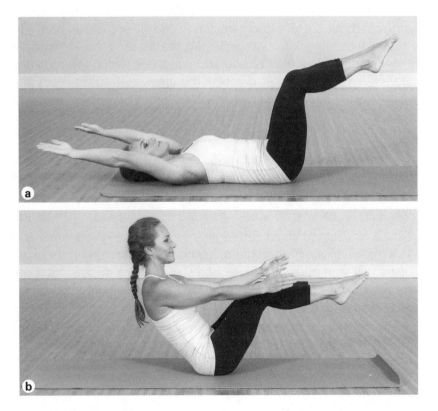

back off the mat *(a)*. Keep the shoulders down and your scapula engaged. This is a move similar to the roll-up.

2. Come all the way up and reach for your toes while keeping your knees bent and legs in tabletop. Exhale on the way up into the movement as the hands reach from the side walls up to your toes as your body lifts *(b)*.

3. Use your abs and the exhalation, not momentum.

4. Inhale at the top to prepare, and then exhale as you roll down, beginning with the lower abs. Using abdominal control, sequentially drop each vertebra down to the mat.

5. As you roll the upper spine down, the arms will travel back to your sides and then overhead. Keep your shoulders down and don't allow the ribs to pop up.

REPETITION

Inhale to prepare and exhale to repeat three more times.

TIP

As your strength increases, aim for a fluid, nonstop rhythm of curl up, roll down.

TEASER

Teaser is more advanced than teaser prep. Just as teaser prep works your spinal extensors and core, so does the full version. It also requires engagement of the hip flexors, quads, adductors, and hamstrings. Ideally you will want to advance to this movement once you have perfected the teaser prep. If you have low back-related injuries, this may not be an ideal exercise for you regardless of how long you have had a Pilates practice. It is always OK to stay with the prep variation or choose another exercise.

TECHNIQUE

1. Lie supine, with your arms at 90 degrees and your legs outstretched flat on the mat *(a)*. To modify, you can begin in the same position as the teaser prep.

2. Inhale to prepare while reaching your arms alongside your ears *(b)*.

3. Exhale as you nod your head slightly while reaching your arms outward to a T-position *(c)*. Remember to scoop your abdominal muscles in and up so that your upper and lower body begin to roll off the mat. Continue to reach your fingertips past your toes and keep your shoulders down so that your body becomes V-shaped.

4. Inhale as you come to the top and open your chest, lifting your head slightly to extend the length of your spine *(d)*.

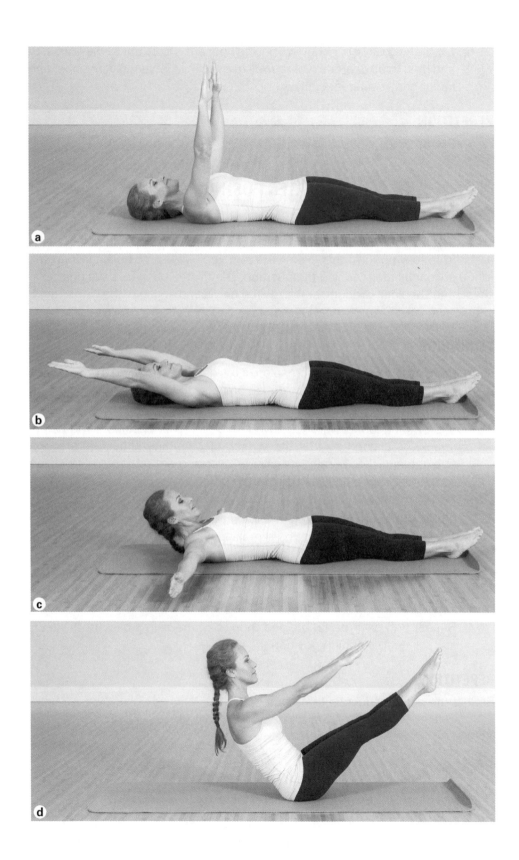

5. Exhale as you roll back down, moving your arms back out to the T-position and then to 90 degrees where they began while lowering your upper and lower body simultaneously.

REPETITION

Repeat three times.

PILATES PUSH-UP

The Pilates push-up is an advanced move. You can start working on it now, but know that it takes a while to build up the core and arm strength and stability required to fully perform this exercise. Work your way up to holding the plank for 60 seconds before adding the push-up. The Pilates push-up develops core, chest, and shoulder strength; stabilizes the pelvis and engages the hamstrings, glutes, and calves.

TECHNIQUE

1. From a standing position, complete a roll-down by following the directions for the standing roll-down exercise on page 147, and place the palms on the mat.
2. Walk the hands forward to move into a high plank position. The hands should be aligned so that the wrists, elbows, and shoulders are in a straight line. The thumbs are aligned with the armpits to create space across the chest, and the palms are spread wide. The heels of the feet should reach toward the back wall to engage the hamstrings and calves *(a)*.
3. Inhale and bend the elbows in toward the midline of the body, lowering the chest toward the mat while making sure that your body, head, and neck all move together so that you are not pulling on your neck and that your back doesn't arch or sink *(b)*. Think of this as a 3-count movement, inhaling as you lower your body toward the floor in three segments and exhale to push up, returning to the plank position.
4. Repeat two or three times, and then walk the palms back to the feet, and roll up to standing position.

REPETITION

Repeat the entire sequence three times.

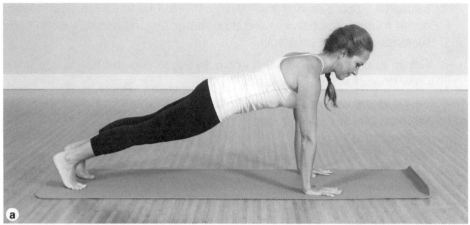

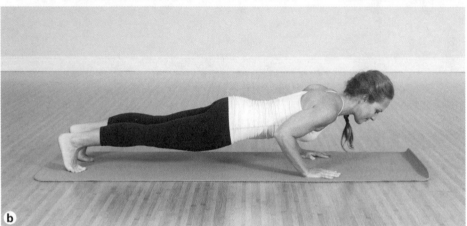

Beginning and End

The standing roll-down can be used at the beginning and end of your workout. It serves as a warm-up exercise before performing other exercises and can be used at the end of your Pilates workout to bring you back into a standing position. The standing roll-down is the perfect exercise for working on your posture.

STANDING ROLL-DOWN

This exercise encourages spinal articulation and abdominal control and can also be used to stretch the back and the hamstrings.

TECHNIQUE

1. Stand tall, with the arms alongside the body, feet are parallel *(a)*.

2. Inhale to prepare, and exhale as you curl the head forward and slowly round through the cervical and then thoracic spine as though the body were peeling itself off a wall.

3. Continue through the lower lumbar spine, letting the hands and arms draw down toward the floor *(b)*.

4. Inhale at the bottom and exhale, rolling back up as you stack each vertebra on top of the other, moving up the imaginary wall until the body is standing tall.

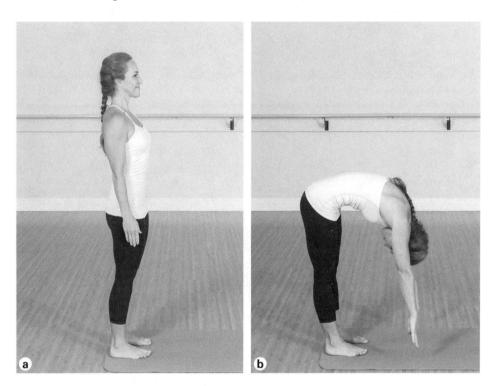

Adding Props to Your Pilates Mat Work

Using props adds an interesting dynamic to your Pilates workout by making the work either harder or easier. While a plethora of props are available, we'll explore three of the easiest to find and use.

Mini Loop Bands

- Place these around your thighs during supine work to help with the tracking of your patella and femur so that your legs and feet don't splay apart.

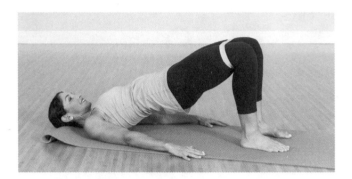

- Place these around your ankles during plank work such as the leg pull front to add resistance and increase the challenge.

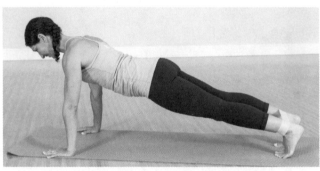

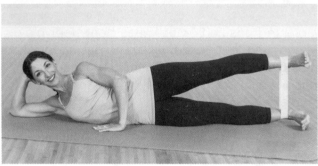

Mini Fitness Ball or Playground Ball

- Hold the 9-inch (23 cm) fitness ball between your thighs to engage your adductors while performing back and core work such as the spine twist.

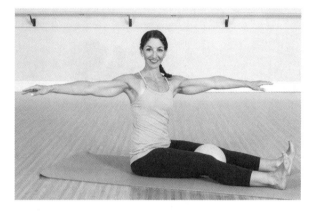

- Hold the ball between your thighs for planks and push-ups to increase adductor work and challenge your core further.

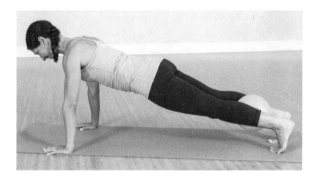

- From a seated position, with knees bent, feet hip-distance apart, heels down, and feet flexed, place the ball at your lower back near your waistband. This will help stabilize your back and increase the challenge of your core work, allowing you to move from slight extension into flexion.

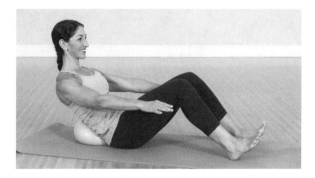

- Squeezing the ball between your hands during supine core work will activate your chest and shoulders.

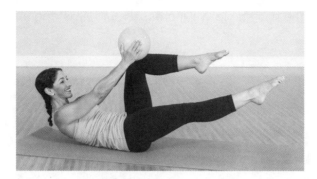

- Placing the ball under your hand during mermaid or saw will increase your range of motion, improving flexibility.

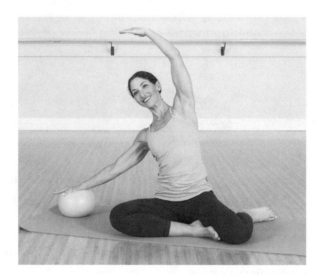

- Squeeze the ball between the ankles during variations of the side-lying leg series and the rollover to challenge stability.

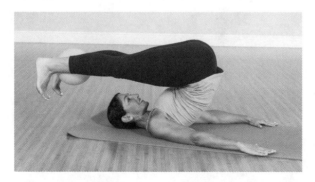

Large Fitness Ball

- Placing your feet on the ball while performing the bridge and working to keep the ball stable will increase your hamstring and glute work.

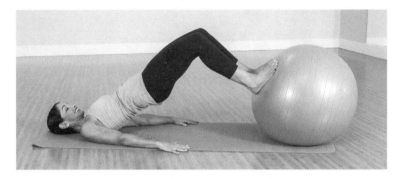

- Once you are in the end position for your bridge, you can press the ball away from your body while maintaining your hip height to add an even greater challenge to your hamstring workout.

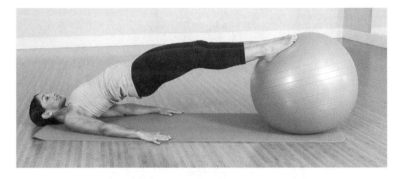

- By lying prone over the ball and working into extension (e.g., swan), you can assist and strengthen your middle and upper thoracic spine while supporting your core.

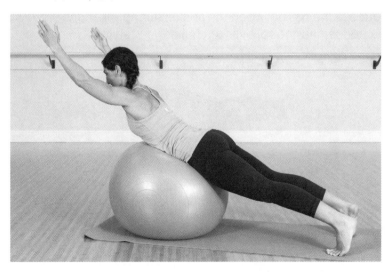

- While in a kneeling position, place the ball next to your body, level with your hip. Use the ball as you move into lateral flexion (e.g., mermaid).

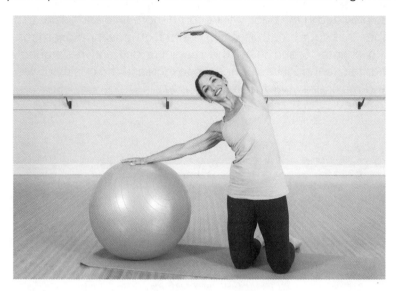

- Increase your push-up challenge by resting your lower legs on a large ball. The closer the ball is to your ankles, the harder the exercise becomes. This is a more advanced move. Only do it if you are confident you can perform it and maintain proper alignment.

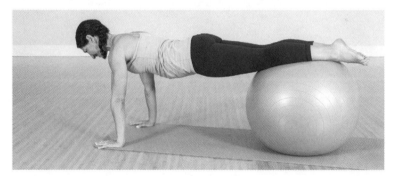

Next Steps

As you progress through your Pilates practice, you will notice that the other exercises provided in the book will become more fluid and easier to perform. Remember that your breath is essential to high-quality movement. As you move into chapter 6 and learn the medicine ball and resistance circuits, remember to use the Pilates principles to increase the quality of your movements and maximize your results.

6 | Training With Medicine Balls and Resistance Bands

Resistance training is not limited to dumbbells and barbells; it may also include medicine balls and resistance bands depending on the goal of the training session. Our athletes often use resistance bands, medicine balls, dumbbells, and barbells all on the same day to cover various aspects of their training.

Resistance Tools and the Seven Pillars

As we discussed in chapter 1, our seven pillars of training include strength, flexibility, mobility, stability, power, speed, and agility. To achieve the greatest success within any of these areas requires not only the proper foundation for movement, but also using the best tools to get there. There is no shortage of props introduced as the newest and greatest tool to improve your strength or flexibility, but in many cases these "newest and greatest" items are fads and not necessary. Don't get us wrong, every now and again something new is created that helps to improve performance, but most people can be successful using just a few tools and props. This chapter teaches you the fundamental movement patterns using medicine balls and resistance bands, which are helpful in developing strength for your Pilates practice as well.

Medicine Balls and Pilates

Pilates develops greater core strength, body awareness, flexibility, and endurance. The benefits of using medicine balls as part of your workout is that they develop all of those key areas. Because you are able to work with bands and balls on a variety of planes, you have the ability to create fluid movement patterns with relative ease. Because no sport occurs in just one plane of movement, we find medicine balls key elements when developing an athlete.

Why Would I Use a Medicine Ball?

The medicine ball has been around for centuries and may be one of the oldest training tools besides heavy rocks. We have heard stories about gladiators using them in their training, and it has been said that the U.S. Military Academy at West Point has included medicine balls in its training for more than 200 years.

Even after all of these years, the medicine ball, or med ball, is still one of the simplest and most effective tools for training. The freedom of movement in many medicine ball exercises replicates movements found in sports and, unlike weights or kettle bells, med balls can be thrown and caught.

What Is a Med Ball?

Not to be confused with the oversized fitness ball, the medicine ball is a solid ball that ranges in weight from 1 pound (.4 kg) to more than 100 pounds (45 kg). It ranges in size from a grapefruit to a beach ball, and textures vary from smooth to grooved.

A ball with a hard shell and air inside will rebound when you throw it into a wall, making it ideal for exercises that develop your reaction time. A "dead ball," on the other hand, has a smooth exterior and will not bounce when you slam it into the ground. It is essentially dead, and more useful for exercises that generate force.

Med Ball Benefits

The most important benefit of using a med ball is, in a word, *power*. Medicine balls are used for throwing and catching drills that help build explosiveness, a characteristic crucial for all athletes. The med ball gives you instant feedback on your power and explosiveness. Medicine ball exercises can also build flexibility and help strengthen your powerhouse.

Incorporating medicine ball training will have a positive effect on your performance by improving cardiovascular fitness, increasing muscular endurance and strength, and fine-tuning speed and power. Incorporating a few of the med ball exercises into your weekly program will round out a pattern of training that prepares you for the field or the court. Always remember, it's the small things within your training that make the biggest difference. Med ball workouts are one of the easiest ways to increase your chances of success because you are able to train from a variety of planes rather than remaining in just a linear plane. Not all sports are created equal, and neither are the movements that they require. Med ball training will prepare your body to perform from all positions.

Selecting a Med Ball

When choosing a medicine ball, first determine whether you need one that bounces or not. Then select one that is heavy enough to create the work you're aiming for, but not so heavy that your form is compromised during the exercise. Very few athletes need to use a ball heavier than 6 pounds (2.7 kg). Remember, you're interested in developing the stabilizing (auxiliary) muscles of the body.

In addition to using a heavier ball, you can increase your output and improve your results by doing the following:

1. Increase the complexity of the movement.
2. Increase movement speeds and intensity of effort.

Coaching Tip

We use medicine ball training to introduce an athlete to our method of resistance training, which focuses on engaging the auxiliary muscles. Our goal is to prevent reliance on only the large muscles to produce movement and instead allow the auxiliary muscles to work and provide stability. For this reason, we usually limit ball weight to 8 pounds (3.6 kg), even when we are training a football lineman.

In 1995 when I first interned with the Chicago Bulls, I dealt primarily with medicine ball throws. Back in those days, Al Vermeil, the head strength coach, invited local kids come to the Berto Center (the former home of the Chicago Bulls) after the pros finished their practice. These kids were athletes trying to get better. They came for strength and speed training, and many were young. The first athlete I worked with was Zach. Zach had a few pounds to lose and needed to develop a strength base. Every day I put him through a medicine ball circuit that was repetitive, but effective. On day one, he had no spatial awareness and could hardly do one squat. After 60 days, he was not only performing the circuit flawlessly, but also doing a 75-percent effort, 50-yard (46 m) tempo run between each throw. He had lost his baby fat. It was time to add an external load, so he started squatting on a balance board, and sure enough Zach nailed it. Not only did he do a flawless squat, but he also maintained a neutral alignment on the balance board. It was a great progression that he worked hard to accomplish. All he knew was that he could squat, but we knew he was able to stabilize positions he couldn't have dreamed of the month before. It was a first step in a long progression that eventually made Zach a dominant football player in high school.

3. Increase acceleration to perform throws with higher intensity.

4. Increase number of repetitions or decrease length of rest periods between sets or both to increase the intensity of an exercise and your training session.

Med Ball Exercises

This medicine ball circuit improves work capacity and strength and allows athletes and clients to train in multiple planes. Athletes can perform the circuit in two ways. 1.) Stand in one place and complete each movement in succession. 2.) Complete a movement, drop the ball, run 20 yards (18 m) out and back, pick up the ball, and do the next movement. The second variation provides more conditioning and offers a way to vary the circuit without changing the overall goal.

This chapter outlines a program consisting of four circuits: two standing circuits, one supine circuit that works the core, and one prone circuit. When executing a med ball circuit, start with the moves that are upright, which focus on the compound movements of your big moves. Some of these use the whole body. After completing the standing exercises, perform the floor exercises.

Ideally, you should complete 20 repetitions of each exercise. Perform 10 repetitions on each side for moves done to both sides. Depending on your level of conditioning, complete at least two rounds of the full four circuits. You can increase the series to 10 rounds, modifying the rest periods as needed.

If you need to modify the program to start, pick five or six exercises, choosing from each circuit. Stick with those exercises for the first few weeks before selecting another group of exercises to work with. Once you're able to perform all of the exercises from each circuit, try the entire program (all exercises in each of the four circuits) for one complete round. When you are able to complete one round, work to increase the number of rounds until you can complete 10 rounds.

Standing Moves: Circuit 1

The medicine ball circuit is loaded with compound movements that require energy from your entire body. Compound exercises require multiple joints and muscle groups and are great movements for a full-body workout. For example, a squat, which is used in several of the following standing movements, involves the quadriceps, hamstrings, and glutes on the lower half of your body, and other exercises use your deltoids, lats, and core on the upper half of your body. In addition to engaging multiple muscle groups, you will also notice the cardiovascular component as your heart rate increases during each of the standing exercises.

BIG CIRCLE

Big circle is the first exercise because it takes you through multiple planes of movement. It engages your entire body, increases your heart rate, and prepares you for the exercises that follow.

TECHNIQUE

1. Start with your feet shoulder-width apart and the medicine ball held above your head with straight arms *(a)*.
2. Swing the ball downward clockwise and create big circles that sweep the floor and then reach to the ceiling *(b)*.
3. As you hit the low spot of this move you should be in squat position with the medicine ball near your shins or ankles and weight distributed equally on both feet and legs *(c)*.
4. After 10 repetitions, perform the circles in a counterclockwise motion.

REPETITION

Perform 20 repetitions. You can determine how many repetitions to do on each side before changing direction; we suggest 10 in one direction and then 10 in the other direction. These 20 movements make up one set.

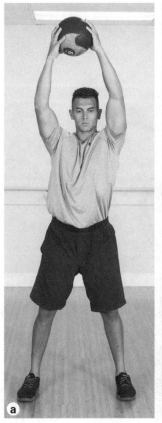
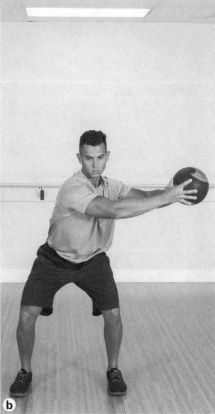
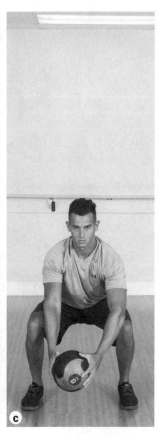

a   b   c

WOOD CHOP

The wood chop movement is straight up and down. Because you're moving from a squat position to standing, your legs and glutes work the entire time. In addition to your lower body, your shoulders, back, and core are active as you lift the ball over your head and lower it with each repetition. Keep the spine neutral and core engaged.

TECHNIQUE

1. Start with your feet shoulder-width apart and the medicine ball held above your head with straight arms *(a)*.
2. Squat as you lower the medicine ball between your legs toward the floor. Your chest is up, back is straight, hips hinge back, and glutes extend past your heels *(b)*.
3. Push through your feet as you return to a standing position, bringing the ball over your head.

REPETITION

Repeat 20 times.

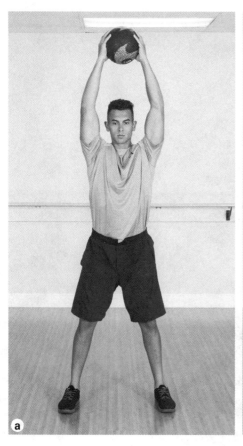
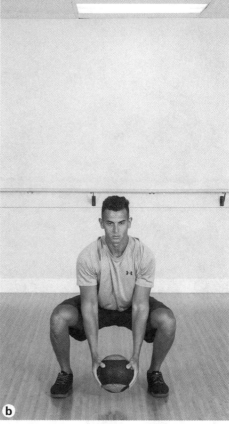

HAMMER THROW

The hammer throw incorporates a squat, but also provides an extension at the top. It's a great way to open the athlete's psoas and quadratus lumborum.

TECHNIQUE

1. Start with the ball between the legs in a squat position. Arms are straight *(a)*.
2. Stand tall with the ball and reach as high as you can over your left shoulder, then return the ball and your body to the start position and repeat, switching from side to side. Elevate the ball high enough to achieve full extension with a bit of rotation *(b)*. This actively stretches the psoas.
3. Complete all repetitions on one side, then switch to the other side. Or alternate from one side to the other side with each repetition.

REPETITION

Complete 10 repetitions on each side.

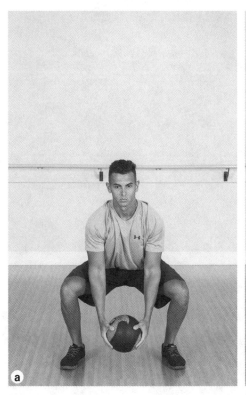
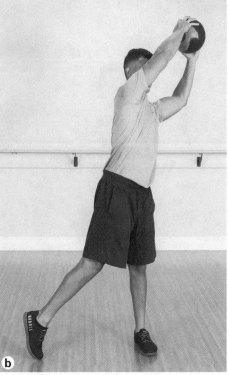

Adding a medicine ball to the squat, reverse lunge, and forward lunge increases the challenge over body-weight exercises because you must recruit additional muscles to provide greater core stability and balance. The following three standing exercises are linked because the location of the med ball is the same for each.

SQUAT

Squatting is the most fundamental movement for building overall strength. This gives the coach and athlete the opportunity to use the same squat throughout their years of training. We use the following glute-dominant squat for our young athletes.

TECHNIQUE

1. Hold the ball to your chest. Feet are either close together or slightly wider than hip distance *(a)*. Squat to your lowest point *(b)*.
2. As you start the squat, hinge the hips slightly back so that the glutes rather than the quads control the movement.
3. Squeeze the glutes to return to standing.
4. To make this move more difficult, extend the medicine ball straight out as you squat and pull it back into your chest as you rise out of the squat.

REPETITION

Repeat 20 times.

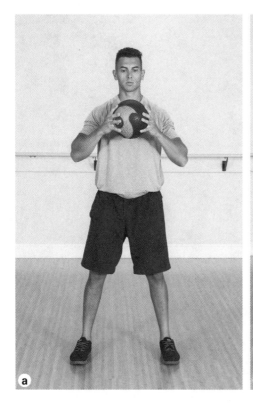
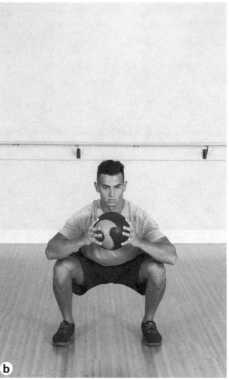

REVERSE LUNGE

The reverse lunge is great for developing an athletic lower body and perfect for any sport requiring speed and power. Think of the reverse lunge as a sport-specific movement. As you return your back leg to a standing position, you should feel your glute and hamstring fire in your front leg. You may also feel a stretch through your back quadriceps while you're in full lunge position.

TECHNIQUE

1. Hold the ball at your chest with both hands *(a)* and take one big step back with your right leg until you are in the bottom of the lunge position.

2. As you lower into the lunge, be sure that your front knee remains directly over your ankle and that your back knee has some bend in it to allow for a full range of motion.

3. Bend your back knee until it is just above the ground *(b)*, then rise all the way up to the starting position.

4. Keep your head upright and your torso straight throughout the lunge.

REPETITION

Complete 10 repetitions on the right side and then 10 on the left. Or alternate right and left legs for a total of 20 repetitions.

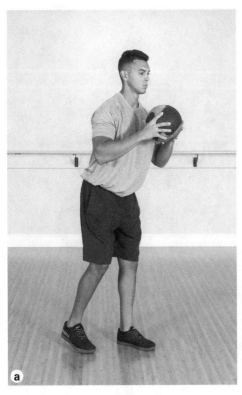
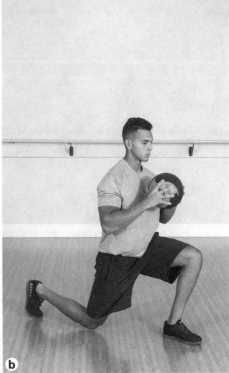

VARIATION

To add a challenge, press the medicine ball from chest height to over your head as you lunge back. Don't use this advanced movement until you can achieve proper form.

FORWARD LUNGE

Lunging creates a unilateral position in which the athlete must stabilize and isolate each leg. The glutes drive the knees and this movement strengthens that pattern. The knee should remain still during lunges. Because success in athletics often depends on how efficiently an athlete can decelerate, be sure to control (decelerate) your body weight and focus on stability.

TECHNIQUE

1. Hold the ball to your chest in both hands *(a)* and take one big step forward until you are in the beginning of the lunge position.
2. Lower your back knee to just above the ground *(b)* and then push off the front heel to return to the starting position.
3. Keep your head up and your torso straight.

REPETITION

Complete 10 repetitions on the right side and then 10 on the left. Or alternate right and left legs for a total of 20 repetitions.

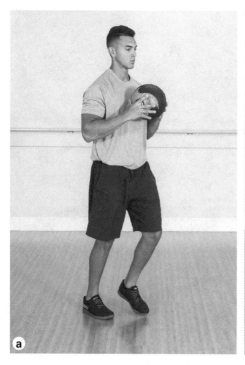
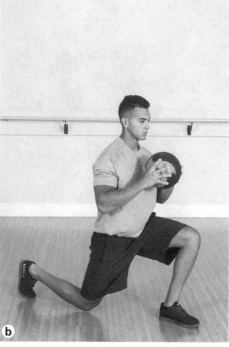

CHEST PASS

The standing chest pass exercise not only develops upper-body strength, but also power, timing, and control. The athlete should absorb the ball coming off the wall (i.e., control the ball when catching it).

TECHNIQUE

1. Hold the ball at chest level in an athletic stance, facing a wall. The feet are slightly wider than hip-distance apart and softly bent. Stand two feet away from the wall, adjusting based on body size, arm length, and the power used to throw the ball *(a)*.
2. Engage the core by keeping the low back stable and navel pulled toward spine.
3. Throw the ball against the wall at chest height and absorb the force as it rebounds back to you *(b)*.
4. Catch it on the rebound, and fire the ball right back to the wall.

REPETITION

Perform 20 repetitions.

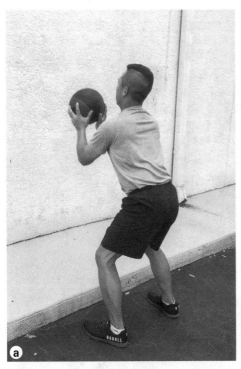
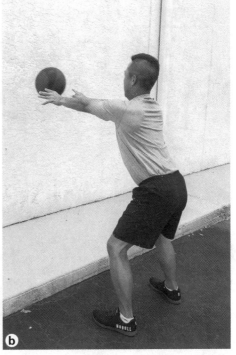

Standing Moves: Circuit 2

Perform the following three exercises as a circuit, completing one set of each and resting as needed between exercises. Complete five rounds, aiming to finish this series as quickly as possible using correct form. Record your total workout time. You can perform this routine at the end of your regular weight-training workout or on its own. As you become more familiar with the circuit, you may be able to decrease the amount of time it takes to perform each round. However, it is better to take your time and use correct form than to rush through these key developmental patterns.

This sequence is ideal for rotational-sport athletes, especially those who play tennis, baseball, softball, or golf. It is important for players of "one-sided sports" to develop a symmetrical strength base. Using a med ball allows for unilateral work in multiple planes without limitations.

OVERHEAD SLAM

The overhead slam recruits the lats and core to develop strength and power. These are necessary for all athletes, but especially those playing rotational sports.

TECHNIQUE

1. Stand with feet shoulder-width apart and hold the ball at arm's length in front of you.

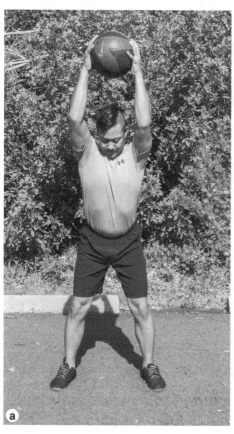 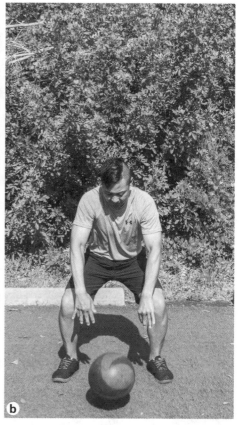

2. Brace your core and raise the ball overhead until you feel a stretch in your abs, but don't bend backward (hyperextend) *(a)*.

3. Slam the ball as hard as you can into the floor *(b)* and catch it on the rebound (or scoop it back up immediately).

REPETITION

Complete 20 repetitions.

ROTATIONAL THROW

Like all rotational exercises, medicine ball rotational throws teach multidirectional movement skills and improve timing and coordination.

TECHNIQUE

1. Begin in a staggered stance, with feet slightly wider than hip-distance apart (imagine a baseball player's batting stance) and hold the ball in both hands. Your right side faces the wall about two feet away. Placing both palms under the ball allows maximum rotation.

2. Twist the torso to your left until you feel a stretch in your core *(a)*, then explosively throw the ball into the wall *(b)*.

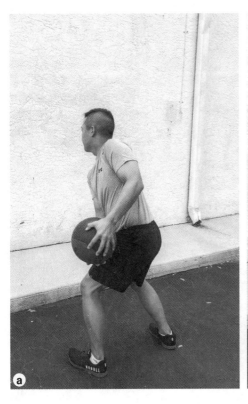
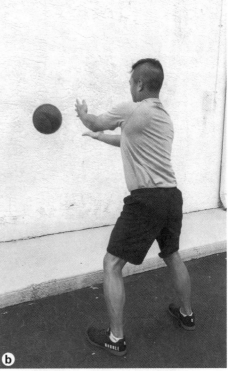

3. Do not allow your feet to pivot or move. Create the movement from the spine, not the hips.

4. Catch the ball and repeat without letting it hit the ground.

REPETITION

Complete 10 throws from one side, then 10 throws on the other side for three sets of 20.

WALL BALL

Wall ball is a power and timing exercise. Because you are going into and coming out of a squat each time you throw the ball against the wall, your quads, glutes, hamstrings, and calf muscles are working throughout the exercise. Timing comes into play because you will throw the ball to the same place on the wall each time.

TECHNIQUE

1. Stand about 12 inches (30 cm) in front of a wall, holding the ball at your chest. Your feet are hip-distance apart in a parallel position. Your knees are softly bent, spine is erect, and core is engaged (a).

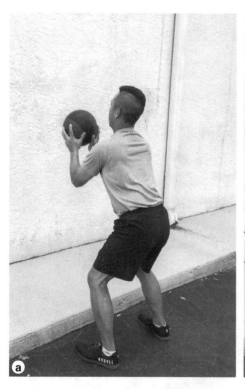
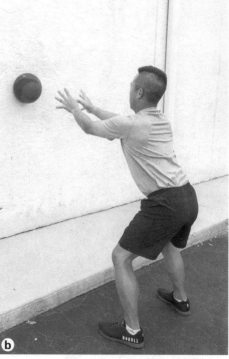

2. Squat, and then as you rise to standing, throw the ball at chest height at a point on the wall above you *(b)*. Do not catch this ball; let it drop and continue. That's one rep. The ball remains at chest level and you're throwing the ball to the wall at the same point for each squat and stand.

REPETITION

Complete 20 repetitions.

Supine Med Ball Core Exercises: Circuit 3

The following core exercises are done from a supine position. By adding the medicine ball to the movement patterns, the athlete learns how to control the movement rather than using momentum. The focus is on using proper form consistently throughout each movement, and the athlete should not feel as if they are whipping the ball around. The additional weight from the ball recruits muscles in the arms, shoulders, chest, and back that would otherwise not be required.

DIAGONAL

Diagonals work the obliques. A cross pattern using the entire torso moves the ball from over one shoulder to between the legs and then over the other shoulder. This movement requires control and quite a bit of shoulder and core strength.

TECHNIQUE

1. Start by lying flat on your back with your knees slightly bent and legs open about hip-distance apart.
2. Press your heels into the floor and pull your toes back toward your face so that your feet are in dorsiflexion.
3. Hold the med ball over your right shoulder next to your ear. The ball is in both hands and both arms are toward one shoulder. The ball may rest on the floor or slightly above it *(a)*. As you roll up and bring the ball between your knees straighten the arms. While the elbows may be soft, the arms are essentially straight.
4. As you exhale, sit up and bring the med ball between your legs to tap the floor *(b)*.
5. Roll back to your starting position, articulating your spine back to the floor. Keep your core engaged throughout the movement.
6. Alternate bringing the ball to the right and left shoulders.

REPETITION

Repeat 10 times on each side.

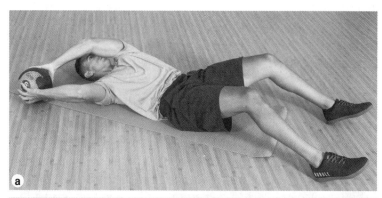

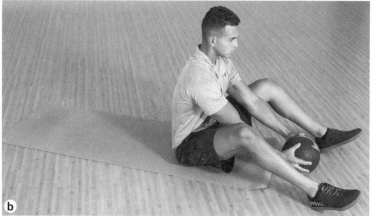

<u>CRUNCH</u>

We have all done crunches before, but adding the medicine ball increases the challenge and recruits additional muscles. Use a 6- to 8-pound (2.7-3.6 kg) medicine ball.

TECHNIQUE

1. Lie on your back and hold the ball above your chest with straight arms. Knees are bent, feet hip-distance apart, and heels pushing into the floor. The toes are pulled back toward your face so that you are in dorsiflexion. Your lower body should remain still throughout the crunches *(a)*.

2. Curl upward until your back is off of the mat. Look at your thighs, and keep a fist-sized space under your chin *(b)*.

REPETITION

Complete 20 repetitions.

TIP

Because this is a crunch and not a full sit-up, you will not rise to an upright position.

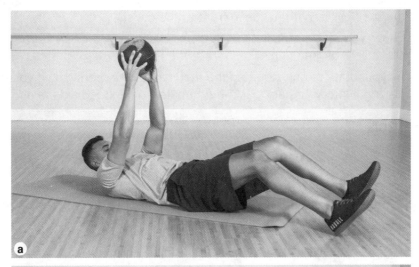

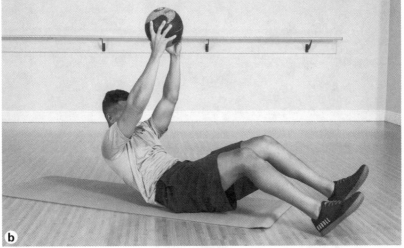

SIDE TAP

Side taps require all of the abdominal muscles to fire together: rectus abdominis and obliques, and when your legs are slightly off the floor, you will notice the transverse abdominals firing too. The trick during this exercise is to make sure that the hip flexors and quads do not take over for the core and do the majority of the work.

TECHNIQUE

1. Begin seated on the floor with knees bent, heels pushing down into the floor, and toes in dorsiflexion. Alternatively, you can lift your feet about 6 inches (15 cm) off the floor without crossing your feet or ankles. Hold the med ball in both hands in front of the chest.

2. Engage your core, and hinge slightly back until your legs and upper body are at a 45-degree angle.

3. As you rotate to one side, tap the med ball on the ground as if you were placing it into your back pocket. Alternate from side to side *(a and b)*.

REPETITION

Repeat 10 times on each side.

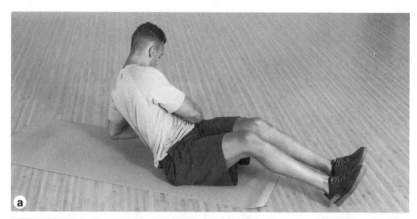

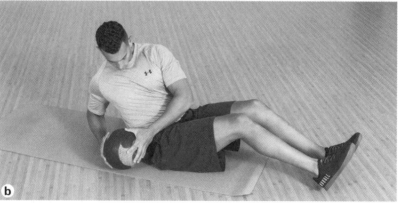

Prone Series: Circuit 4

Working in the prone position challenges your mid- and upper-thoracic muscles and improves your extension. It's the perfect counterbalance for sports that pull the body forward and require rotation. All athletes will benefit from developing greater strength and flexibility throughout their middle and upper back.

SUPERHERO TAP

Going into extension from a prone position requires a combination of mid-thoracic strength and flexibility. The weight of the medicine ball increases the challenge and recruits additional shoulder and upper-back muscles. Maintaining proper shoulder position prevents the trapezius from doing all of the work.

TECHNIQUE

1. Lie facedown with the ball extended in front of you and legs extended toward the wall behind you. The navel is pulled in toward the spine, hips are pressed into the floor, and the tailbone reaches down toward the heels *(a)*.

2. Inhale to prepare, and exhale to peel your chest up from the floor until you feel your midback engage. Inhale to prepare, and exhale as you lift your legs 4 to 6 inches (10-15 cm) off the floor. Keep your core engaged and hips pressing into the floor *(b)*.

3. Tap the med ball from side to side while maintaining the contraction in your middle and upper-thoracic spine (not your lumbar, or lower, spine).

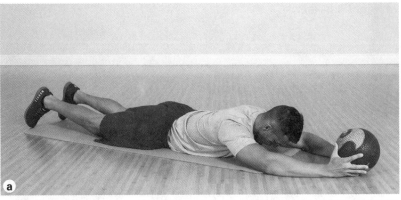

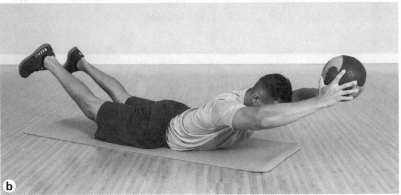

REPETITION

Alternate tapping the ball from one side to the other 20 times.

TIPS

- This move should look like the up position in a Superman while tapping the medicine ball in front of you from side to side.
- Always inhale as you prepare for your movement and exhale to execute.

PLANK

Plank is an ideal core stabilizer that also engages your chest, shoulders, upper back, glutes, and legs. Work to hold each plank for a minimum of 30 seconds.

TECHNIQUE

1. Begin in a plank position with your toes on the floor hip-distance apart and your heels pressing back toward the wall behind you. Place the med ball under one palm and make sure your hand and wrist are aligned under your shoulder. Your wrist, elbow, and shoulder on the other arm form a straight line *(a)*.

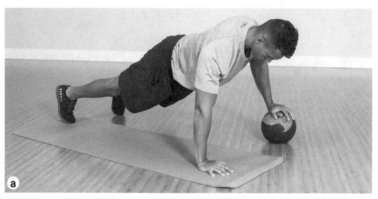

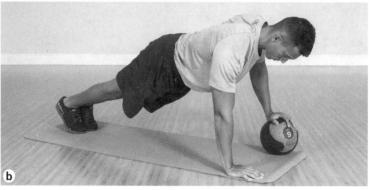

REPETITION

After 30 seconds on one side, roll the ball to the other side and hold for 30 seconds.

TIPS

For additional challenge, try these variations.

1. Keep your legs close together to narrow your base of support *(b)*.
2. Lift one foot off the floor, keeping the pelvis level. Holding for 15 to 30 seconds, then switch legs.

ONE-ARMED PUSH-UP

Push-ups incorporate a variety of muscles within just one exercise. You can change the muscle focus slightly by using either a full push-up position or a kneeling position or by adjusting your hand placement. Placing the medicine ball under one hand increases instability, which requires more use of chest, shoulder, and core muscles to maintain the correct form.

TECHNIQUE

1. Get into a push-up position with one hand on the ball, making sure the wrist, elbow, and shoulder of the other arm are in a straight line *(a)*. The med ball should be slightly off to the side to create more space in order to lower to the floor easier.

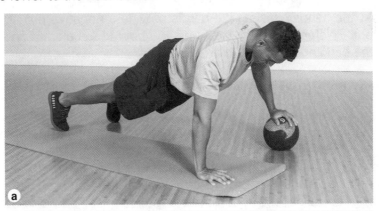

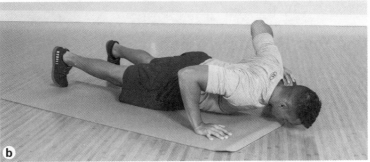

2. Lower your chest toward the floor *(b)* and then push up. At the top, roll the ball to the other hand.

REPETITION

Complete five repetitions on each side.

VARIATION

For an additional challenge, perform the push-ups explosively so that your hand rises off the ball and you switch hands in midair, landing on the ball before you lower into the next push-up.

Once you have completed the first round of the medicine ball circuit, you will have completed 16 exercises and nearly 300 repetitions. Each move is done for 20 repetitions, and there are 10 exercises in this group. You can complete this circuit as many times as you deem necessary to reach your goals.

Resistance Bands and Pilates

Resistance bands are useful tools that increase the strength of your muscles and stimulate growth; however, they are sometimes overlooked for strength training. Many people love to grab the heavy barbells and dumbbells, but it's important to remember that resistance bands are an important part of your training toolbox. Because resistance bands challenge your muscles by creating resistance in multiple directions, you can create a full-body workout using just the bands. Resistance bands provide a negative pull after each movement. This eccentric pull teaches you how to decelerate and how to control the band and the pattern.

Resistance Band Benefits

One of the biggest benefits of a resistance band workout is that bands allow the full range of motion, working many parts of a muscle often not worked by free weights. This allows you to perform more controlled movements, keep constant tension on the muscles, and emphasize both the concentric and eccentric portions of the movement. Resistance bands are lightweight, travel easily, and allow you to complete a varied resistance workout without having to be in the gym.

Selecting Your Resistance Band

Selecting the correct resistance band is as important as selecting the correct dumbbell for each exercise. You should be able to complete 10 repetitions of whatever exercise you are doing with correct form and alignment; however, by number 10 you should feel as if your muscles have been working and are slightly fatigued. If you are breezing through your movements, choose a more challenging band.

Each brand of resistance bands is slightly different. Generally, colors indicate the resistance levels. At Beyond Motion, we use the Slastix brand. Each band has plastic handles and a protective sleeve over the elastic tubing. The colors and resistances are as follows: Yellow is the lightest, red is medium, blue is heavy, and green is extra heavy. For athletes over 6-feet (1.8 m) tall, longer bands may be required for certain exercises in order to maintain correct form and range of motion.

To make a strength workout more difficult, you can make a resistance band exercise more challenging in several ways:

1. Use a band with a higher resistance level.

2. Use two bands at once, combining levels to achieve the resistance you want.

3. If you are standing on the band, widen your stance to create greater resistance in the band.

4. To change the focus of the exercise, release some of the resistance and perform the exercise with greater speed to improve endurance and timing.

Resistance Band Exercises

Sport-specific conditioning focuses on improving movement patterns rather than training individual muscle groups. The versatility of resistance band exercises allows an athlete to mirror the movement patterns of their sport using varying degrees of resistance. Bands play an important role in injury prevention and rehabilitation. Athletes can also incorporate these exercises

Rick's Tips

Over the course of my coaching career, some of my methods have changed. The biggest change I've made is scheduling athletes' resistance band workouts for days they don't lift weights. This allows us to focus on refining positions and training the smaller muscles that contribute to a movement. We can also test their cardiovascular capacity by creating volume. Resistance band training gets the athlete out of their comfort zone. Athletes love the variety this type of training brings. Although they might dread it at first because of the number of reps they do for each exercise, when they are done with the workout, they love the way their bodies feel. They feel fatigue, but without too much muscle breakdown.

Because resistance bands are easier on the joints than dumbbells, this type of training can be ideal for in-season athletes. For example, by adding resistance from a band during a squat or split squat, an athlete can develop greater depth and range of motion during the movement. Using multiple variations of the most common conditioning exercises allows the body to recruit additional muscles. When exercises are done under a load, form can deteriorate because of compensation and instability. Therefore, doing the same exercise with a resistance band brings the athlete back to ground zero: It makes their body remember the correct pattern and provides a chance to work on stability.

into an off-season training program, when recovery and regeneration are important.

When using resistance bands for strength or general training, it's important to select the most appropriate resistance level. Bands are typically available in tube and loop styles. Tube bands have handles and are ideal for the following strength-training exercises.

SQUAT

Adding the resistance band to a body-weight squat increases the challenge as you return to the standing position. You are working against the resistance while maintaining a more vertical posture. You can increase the resistance by using a slightly wider stance or by using a heavier band.

TECHNIQUE

1. Stand on the resistance band with both feet. Feet are shoulder-width apart.
2. Hold the resistance band handles at shoulder level with your palms facing forward *(a)*. (The band should be behind your arms rather than in front of your body.)

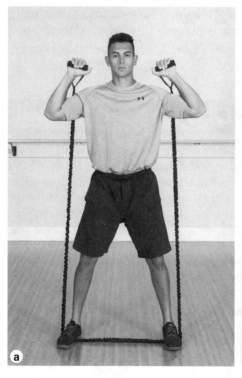
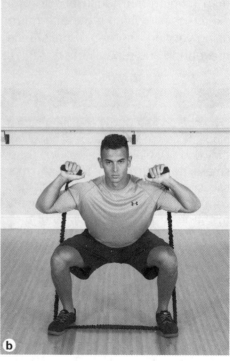

3. Lower into a full squat while maintaining the band at shoulder height *(b)*.

4. Return to the starting position.

REPETITION

Complete 20 repetitions.

SPLIT SQUAT

Just as in the resistance band squat, using a resistance band during a body-weight split squat increases the workload as you return to the starting position.

TECHNIQUE

1. Stand with the feet hip-width apart and a resistance band under the left foot. Step the right foot back approximately 2 feet (.6 m), and balance on the ball of the foot. The head and back are straight and in a neutral position *(a)*.

2. Lower the body into a lunge by bending at the left hip and knee until the thigh is parallel to the floor and the back knee is as close to the floor as possible. The body should follow a straight line down toward the floor *(b)*.

3. Return to the starting position.

REPETITION

Complete four sets of 10 repetitions on each leg.

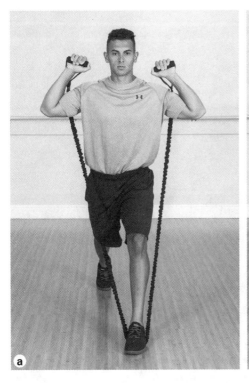
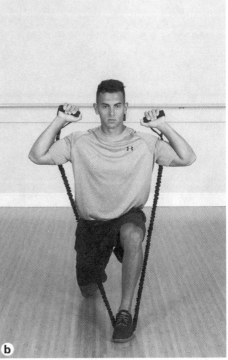

BENT-OVER ROW

Bent-over rows work the lats, middle and lower-thoracic spine, and core and to a degree the biceps. The benefit of using the band is that you can alter your hand and arm position and the height of your elbows to create slight variations all while maintaining the same body alignment. This is one of our favorites. It's one of the best scapular exercises because it lets you engage your entire body with the lighter load.

TECHNIQUE

1. Stand with the feet at least hip-distance apart and a resistance band under the arch of each foot. Hold the handles, or slightly below the handles, and make an X with the bands.
2. Hinge forward from the hips until you reach a 45-degree angle. Keep your neck long, eyes down, and shoulders relaxed and away from your ears *(a)*.
3. Pull the bands up toward your waist, keeping your elbows in toward your body while reaching them toward the back wall. Squeeze your shoulder blades down and in when performing the rowing motion *(b)*.

REPETITION

Perform four sets of 20 repetitions each.

TIP

You may increase the resistance by holding the bands lower than the handles or by stepping your feet wider apart.

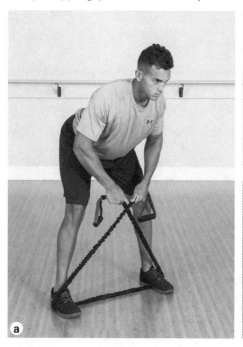

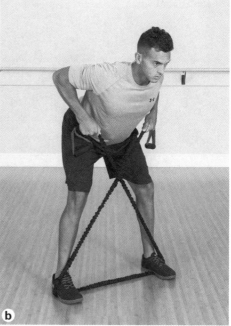

DIAGONAL WOOD CHOP

Adding the resistance band under your feet will increase the resistance as you move through the full range of motion and decrease resistance as you return to your starting position. You can increase or decrease the resistance by changing the placement of your feet. You can also play with the tempo safely without relying on momentum. Wood chops with a resistance band work many muscles at once. Your shoulders, abs, obliques, glutes, quads, lower back, upper back, hamstrings, abductors, and adductors are all engaged throughout the exercise. This is a great exercise for anyone, and especially for athletes who play rotational sports.

TECHNIQUE

1. Stand with your feet about hip-distance apart and your left foot on slightly less than half of the band. One handle is on the floor close to your left foot. Hold the other handle in both hands (or slightly below the handle).

2. Lower into a squat and bring the handle you're holding down toward your right ankle *(a)*. As you stand up, bring that handle toward your left shoulder, creating a diagonal line across the front of your body *(b)*.

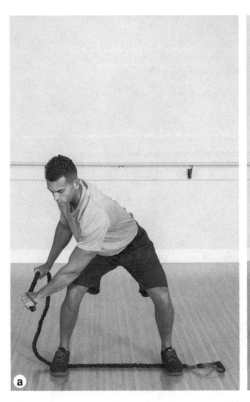
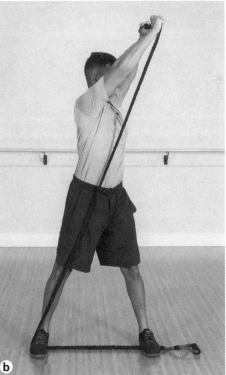

3. During this motion, your feet are stationary and you rotate through the trunk.

4. Return back to your starting position and repeat.

REPETITION

Perform four sets of 10 repetitions, alternating sides between sets.

HIGH ROW

By using the band, you should be able to fully engage your rhomboids and lats without squeezing your traps and concentrate on the retraction instead of on moving a heavy weight. This should make it possible to execute the row with greater ease, making the action feel simple although not easy.

TECHNIQUE

1. Stand with feet hip-distance apart and feet on a resistance band. The knees are slightly bent.

2. Cross the band to create an X. Hold the handles, or slightly below the handles for greater resistance. Your arms should hang in front of your thighs, palms facing your body *(a)*.

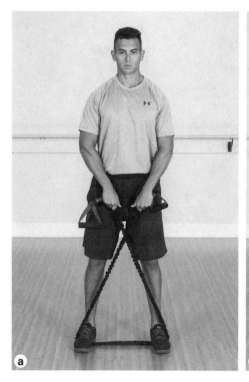 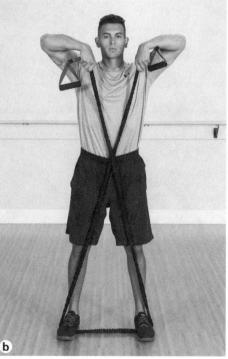

3. Pull the elbows up so your hands are at the height and width of your shoulders, pinching your shoulder blades inward toward your spine. Maintain a relaxed neck and traps *(b)*.

4. Return to the start position. When you bend the elbows into a high pull position and they are reaching outward to the side walls, the scapulae pinch toward the spine and the elbows are essentially in alignment with the medial delt.

REPETITION

Complete 20 repetitions.

BICEPS CURL

Control the contraction with a smooth movement from start to end. Work to find resistance at both ends of the movement.

TECHNIQUE

1. Stand with the feet shoulder-width apart, a band placed under the arches of the feet. For less resistance, place only one foot on the center of the band.

2. Hold the handles with an underhand grip (palms facing up). The arms hang at your sides, with the elbows tucked close to your sides. Maintain the elbow position throughout the exercise *(a)*.

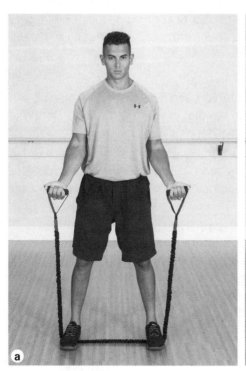
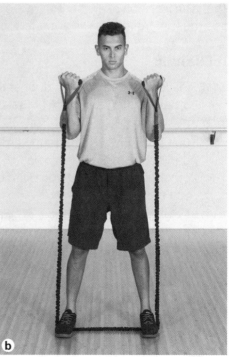

3. Flex at the elbows and curl the band up to approximately shoulder level. You do not need to touch your shoulder to complete the curl *(b)*.

4. Return to the starting position in a controlled manner.

5. The shorter the length of the band on either side of you, the more difficult the exercise is.

REPETITION

Complete four sets of 20 curls. You can do 20 on one side and change hands to repeat 20 on the other. Repeat four sets.

TIPS

- Keep your back and head straight and core engaged throughout the movement.
- Keep your shoulders still to avoid engaging your trapezius, and flex only the elbow.

VARIATIONS

- For unilateral work, alternate curling one arm at a time, completing 10 repetitions on each side.
- Perform a reverse curl by gripping the band with the palms facing the floor.

TRICEPS EXTENSION

This is an isolation exercise: The movement occurs at only one joint and targets one muscle group, allowing you to focus your efforts on your triceps muscles.

TECHNIQUE

1. Place your band on the floor and step on one side of it while holding the other handle, or slightly below the handle, in your right hand.

2. Extend your arm to the sky *(a)* and then allow your elbow to bend so that it is pointing as far upward to the sky as you can and your hand is down towards your scapula *(b)*. The band will hang down your back. Your other hand can be at your side or across your abdominals to make sure you maintain a tight core.

3. Extend the elbows until your arms are fully extended.

4. Return to the starting position in a controlled manner.

REPETITION

Complete four sets 20 repetitions. When you change to the other arm, you should follow the same instructions. The top arm is the one working the triceps.

TIPS

- Stay tall and keep your shoulders relaxed.
- If you have a frozen shoulder, you will not be able to get into this position. If immobility is a factor, shorten or change the range of motion. The tighter you are in your traps and pecs, the less likely you are to get your elbow directly upward to a 90 degree angle, but try to make this your goal.

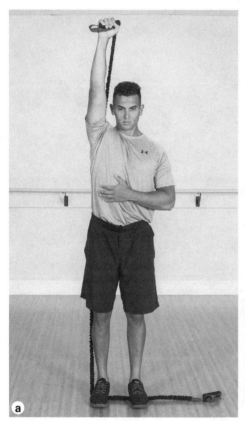 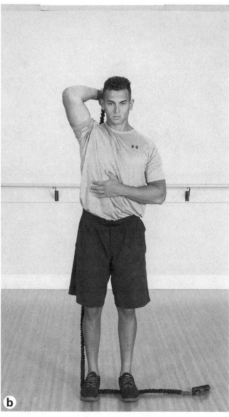

CHEST PRESS

The chest press tones and strengthens the muscles in your arms and chest.

TECHNIQUE

1. Stand with your feet about hip-distance apart. Wrap the resistance band around your chest from front to back and bring the handles back to the front of your body. Hold the handles at chest height with your thumbs near your armpits and elbows pointing toward the floor *(a)*.
2. Keep your knees slightly bent and as you exhale, press the handles out in front of you *(b)*.
3. Return to the starting position in a controlled manner.

REPETITION

Complete 20 repetitions.

VARIATION

In addition to performing the exercise bilaterally (both sides at the same time), you can also perform the chest press unilaterally (one side at a time).

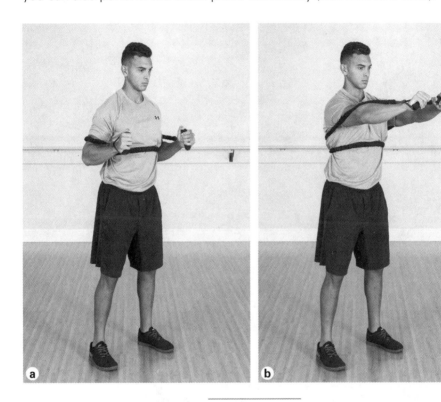

For all of you cyclists, triathletes, runners, and swimmers, the following exercises are dedicated to you. They counteract the sense of being pulled forward that comes from having a tight chest and weak and rounded shoulders and upper back. These three exercises are key to strengthening your upper back, opening your chest, and improving your posture.

REVERSE FLY

The resistance band reverse fly works the upper back and shoulders. It's a great exercise not only for developing greater strength, but also improving posture and body awareness.

TECHNIQUE

1. Stand with your feet about hip-distance apart. Loop the band around your hands to create additional resistance. Hands are about shoulder-width apart.
2. Raise your arms straight out in front of you at about shoulder height *(a)*. Open the arms to the side, pulling on the band, pinching the shoulder blades together, and opening your chest *(b)*.
3. Return arms to starting position but don't allow slack in the band. Keep some resistance throughout.

REPETITION

Complete four sets of 20 repetitions.

TIP

Keep your shoulders relaxed and your arms straight the entire time; if you have trouble keeping them straight, try a lighter band.

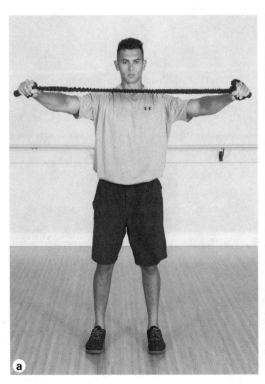
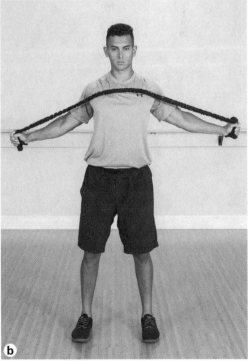

SCAPTION

Scaption exercises strengthen several muscles in your shoulders and back. Think of it as the retraction of your shoulder blades. This exercise is commonly used in the prevention and rehabilitation of rotator cuff injuries, and one we use often with athletes of all ages.

TECHNIQUE

1. Stand with your feet about hip-distance apart. Place one handle in each hand and wrap the band around your palms to create greater resistance.
2. Hold the arms in front of your body with your hands above your head (a).
3. Maintain straight elbows as you pull the hands apart, retracting your shoulder blades and feeling the pinch as they move toward your spine *(b)*.
4. Return to the starting position in a controlled manner. The starting position creates neutrality in the scapula. As you begin, the scaption will naturally occur.

REPETITION

Complete four sets of 20 repetitions each.

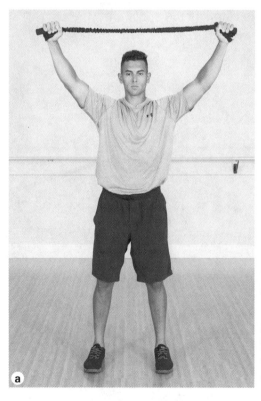
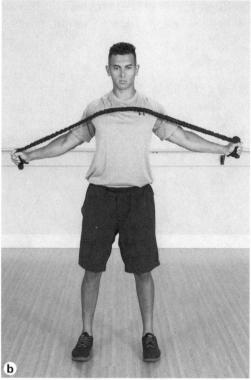

TIP

Keep the torso straight, head up, and shoulders relaxed during the exercise. The trapezius should not be the main mover; rather focus on the rhomboids and opening your chest.

OVERHEAD PRESS

The overhead press strengthens the shoulder muscles and increases stability in the body. Pressing against the resistance of the band upward is done with the shoulder or deltoid muscles.

TECHNIQUE

1. Stand with both feet on the center of the band, hip-width apart.
2. Bring the handle of the band above the shoulder so that elbow is bent 90 degrees *(a)*.
3. Press the arm straight up, keeping the shoulder down *(b)*. Slowly lower the handle to the starting position.

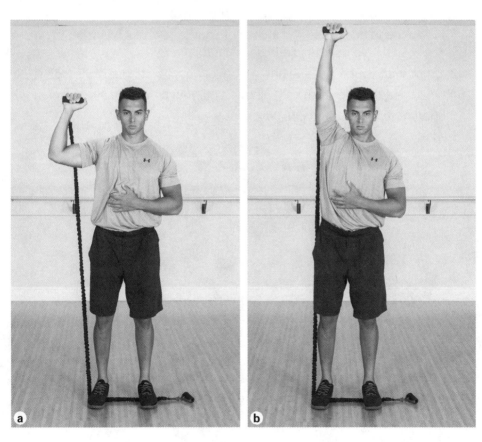

REPETITION

Complete four sets of 10 repetitions. When you change to the other arm, you should follow the same instructions.

TIPS

- Keep your abdominals pulled in tight, and slightly bend your knees.
- If the band is too tight to fully extend your arms, stand on the center of the band with one foot instead of two. This will give the band a bit more length.

SEATED ROW

The seated row with a resistance band works your middle and upper back. From your lats to your rhomboids and the middle and lower trapezius, most of your major back muscles are working.

TECHNIQUE

1. Sit on the floor with your legs slightly bent in front of you.
2. Loop the band around the arches of your feet, cross it in front of you in an X, and hold one handle in each hand.
3. Start with your arms straight in front of you, pointing at your toes *(a)*.
4. Pull the arms back with bent elbows until your hands touch your chest *(b)*.
5. Return to the starting position.

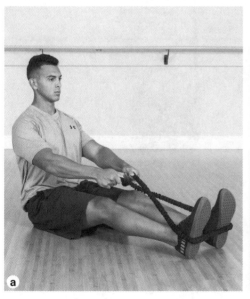
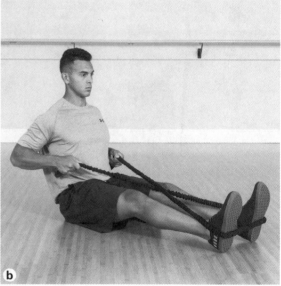

REPETITION

Complete four sets of 20 repetitions.

VARIATIONS

You may perform this exercise two ways:

- Grab the handles with the palms facing inward toward each other so that your elbows reach below your rib cage as you pull them back.
- Grab the handles with the palms facing the floor.

PUSH-UP

Push-ups are a great body-weight exercise that strengthen all the muscles of your upper body. The band's greatest benefit is to make the push-up more difficult.

TECHNIQUE

1. Place the band so that the center of it is on your back and your hands are holding the handles in front of you. The band is under your armpits.
2. Get into the bottom of a push-up position while holding one handle in each hand. The hands are flat on the floor. The band should be pulled tight at the lowest point of the push-up *(a)*.

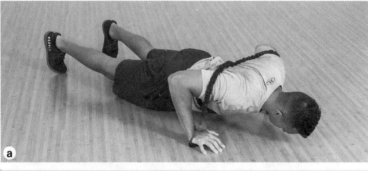

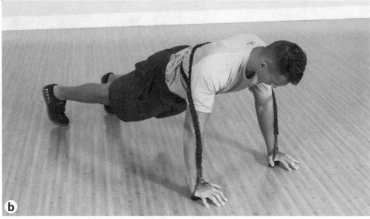

3. Push yourself up until your arms are fully extended *(b)*, then slowly lower back to the original position.

REPETITION

Complete four sets of 10 repetitions.

_____

Using both med balls and bands in the first training microcycle is a great way to evaluate your progress. Because of the low load, this equipment gives you a chance to see exactly which movements need to be addressed. We are always evaluating to see how we can coach better in order to get the athlete to perform better. This process evolves during an athlete's training. Scheduling a med ball circuit and band circuit during the first week of training provides vital information about an athlete's limitations and strengths both physical and mental. This allows us to develop the best training plan for that athlete.

Assessing performance levels is not a one-time event, but rather an ongoing process. When you write a program, it becomes the athlete's game plan. Although the first few workouts are scripted, you have to be ready to pivot based on what you see during their subsequent training sessions. Experience helps a coach develop this talent, and young coaches should not get caught up in sticking to the plan if their athlete is performing under or beyond expectations. I was taught early on that the first two weeks are an evolution of consistently changing programs. One size does not fit all and you should be ready to format a program that is specific to the needs of the athlete. Short-term remedies give you short-term results. It is important to teach the athlete that each day is built from the last day, and progressions are a process and take time. I tell all of our athletes, "I want you to leave this session feeling worked and your body taxed, but making progress. My job is not to empty the tank; my job is to fill it up so it has the fuel for you to come in and train the next day."

Next Steps

Once your athlete develops a strong foundation from the med ball and resistance band workouts, it's time for them to progress onto dumbbell and barbell training. As we mentioned previously, everyone takes a different training path to meet their goals. When dealing with much younger athletes or athletes with little weight room experience, give them time to learn their foundational movement patterns before moving them onto the next phase. This could take weeks, or it could take months. It is more important to focus on the form and function of each movement than on how quickly someone moves from one progression to another.

Chapter 7 takes you through the intricacies of dumbbell and barbell training, which are effective ways to develop the strength needed for optimal athletic performance. Read each section carefully so that you are familiar with all of the exercises and the set-up for each one. Athletes will begin with lighter weight until they understand the movement pattern and are able to execute it flawlessly before increasing the weight.

7 Fundamental Strength Exercises

When developing an athlete for sport or reconditioning an athlete from injury, we use a variety of modalities to safely prepare them for competition. Two of the primary pieces of equipment we use are dumbbells and barbells. Both are effective for building strength, and each has its own advantages. Dumbbells allow the athlete to do many unilateral movements (movements on one side of the body), which create balance. They also allow the athlete to learn a movement pattern for a particular exercise while recruiting stabilizing muscles. In essence, dumbbells provide motor pattern learning using external weights. Barbells, on the other hand, are our primary tool for compound movements once athletes have adapted to a reasonable load and are able to control their body, the patterns, and the weights. Barbells are unmatched when an athlete is trying to develop strength and power. They allow us to add optimal loads, which allows us to build the strength and power needed to be an effective athlete.

Training With Dumbbells

Dumbbells accommodate movement on a variety of planes and allow you to work through a free range of motion without restriction. They can be used for single or multiple planes of movement. Dumbbells allow you to work each side individually, alternately, or simultaneously. Single-sided exercises can correct muscle imbalances and asymmetries. By incorporating corrective exercises with dumbbells, you can target specific deficiencies and decrease the risk of injury.

The farther you hold the dumbbells from your center, the more stability you must generate to control the load.

If you're lacking stability, you will not be able to control the load. With a dumbbell, the farthest you can move the weight is an arm's length away, allowing you more control depending on the load.

With so many types of exercises available, it can be difficult to know where to start and how to progress. Using heavy weights too soon can cause poor form, which can then lead to injury. Start by selecting a weight at which you can do a maximum of 10 repetitions. Your ninth or 10th repetition should feel like work, but without strain. As the last reps become easier, increase your overall weight for that exercise, but make sure that as you increase your weight, you do not sacrifice your form.

Safety above all else is paramount. Not only do you want to make sure that you are fit enough to use these programs, but also that you are ready mentally and physically to train in a safe and effective manner. Selecting equipment (bands, medicine balls, dumbbells, barbells) that is appropriate for your current skill and strength level is the most important consideration. Ideally, your training space should be free of distractions and items that could prevent you from properly setting up and completing your exercises. We prefer that you train with a partner or spotter so that someone is available to assist you with your heavier weights as needed. If you do not have someone available to train with at the gym, ask someone who works at the facility if you can "have a spot." There's probably a trainer that can help you with your heavier sets. If you are at home and no one is available to help you, it is best to maintain moderate weights that you have complete control over.

In a pinch, a Smith machine can replace a barbell and squat stand. A Smith machine is a large piece of equipment available at most big-box gyms that provides support and assistance for barbell work. A base and side rails support the bar and assist you with the amount of weight you are using.

Dumbbell Exercises

We start with dumbbells because it's a great way to introduce strength training to an athlete. You are creating patterns that require stability, strength, and precision. Athletes love to compensate, and this is a great opportunity to reinforce the proper movement.

DUMBBELL SQUAT

The dumbbell squat is an introductory exercise that provides the athlete with immediate feedback from the body.

TECHNIQUE

1. Stand with your feet just wider than shoulder width and toes turned slightly outward.

2. Hold one dumbbell in each hand. The palms face forward and elbows align with the ribcage. Make sure the weights are not resting on your shoulders but are slightly above *(a)*.

3. Begin the downward (or eccentric) phase of the squat by hinging your hips back and lowering your backside as if you were sitting into a chair.

4. Keep your core engaged and your thoracic spine stable. Work to keep the dumbbells in the same position with the spine long to prevent rounding of the back *(b)*.

5. Push through your heels as you begin the ascent, or the concentric phase, back to the starting position.

REPETITION

Complete 10 repetitions.

TIPS

- Keep the feet planted on the floor and do not rise onto your toes. This ensures that the glutes do the work rather than the quads.
- Keep your chest lifted and don't let your torso cave forward, which increases the strain on the lower back; pull your navel toward your spine.

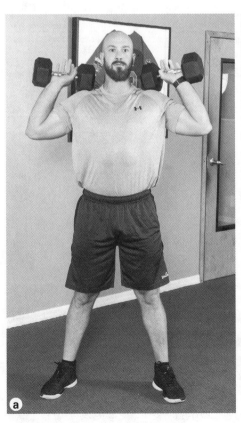 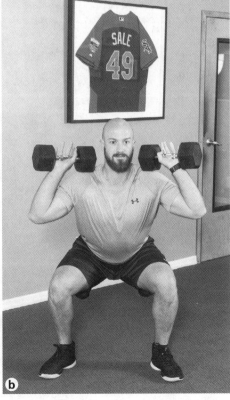

DUMBBELL ROMANIAN DEADLIFT

The dumbbell RDL creates a hip hinge and a tight thoracic spine. You're looking for the mid-thoracic to be completely engaged and tight (but not tight as in muscle soreness and tightness). It's also a great way to uncover deficiencies. For instance, tight hamstrings limit the range of motion of the RDL.

TECHNIQUE

1. Stand with your feet about hip-distance apart, toes pointing directly forward. Hold the dumbbells in front of your thighs, with your palms facing you *(a)*.

2. Bend your knees slightly to increase mobility on the downward phase. Before you begin your descent, engage your core and set your back into the thoracic arch position. The best way to establish your thoracic arch is to begin by slightly hinging at your hips so that as your torso moves forward, your glutes shift slightly back. Keep your chest up and shoulders wide so that you feel engagement in your middle and upper thoracic spine. As you lower the weights toward your knees, you should feel not only your core and midback engage, but also feel a hamstring stretch.

3. As you hinge at the hips to lower your upper body toward the floor, push your glutes behind you and keep the dumbbells close to your legs. Think about pressing your backside against a wall to ensure your hips are following the correct path *(b)*.

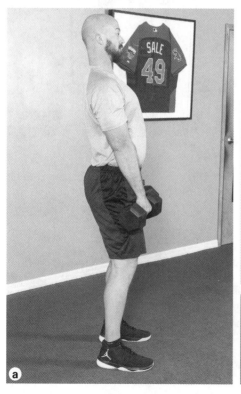
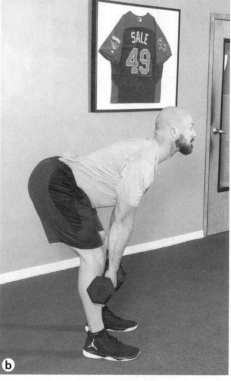

4. Return to the start position by slowly dragging the dumbbells back up your legs and hinge up. Pull your knees back as you rise and do not pull your back up first; that will put a strain on your lower back.

REPETITION

Complete 10 repetitions.

TIPS

- Keep your shoulders back and your chest open and wide to ensure a stable thoracic spine and proper posture.
- Look forward rather than down at the ground.
- When you feel your back starting to round, stop; that is your depth for your RDL. As your flexibility, mobility, and strength increase, your depth will increase as well.

DUMBBELL ROW

The dumbbell row is a great back developer. It's important to teach scapular retraction early so the athlete does not engage the traps during the exercise. An effective cue is to tell athletes to pinch their scapula down and in toward the spine.

TECHNIQUE

1. Stand with your feet hip-distance apart, with a slight bend in the knees. Hinge the upper body forward from the hips at about a 45-degree angle.

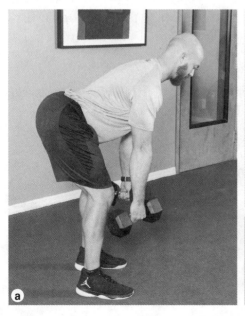 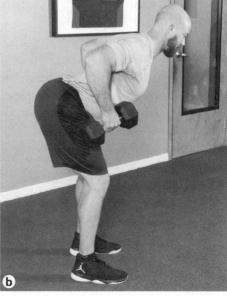

2. Hold a dumbbell in each hand, with arms extended. Choose from three grips for this exercise: overhand (pronated) with palms facing toward you, underhand (supinated) with palms facing away from you, or a neutral grip with your palms facing each other. Keep your chest lifted, back muscles engaged, and a thoracic arch in the back *(a)*.

3. Pull the dumbbells up and back toward your chest (not your chin); think about squeezing the middle section of your back and your shoulder blades together rather than pulling up with your traps *(b)*.

4. Slowly lower the dumbbells with control to the start position.

REPETITION

Complete 10 repetitions.

DUMBBELL REVERSE LUNGE

This exercise isolates the glutes. The glutes are tonic muscles that need to be turned on so the hamstrings and quads don't take over and movement. Concentrate on engaging and feeling the glutes during this exercise so that the hamstrings and quads don't overtake the movement.

TECHNIQUE

1. From a standing position, hold a dumbbell in each hand by your sides *(a)* and take a big step back with the left foot. This step is big enough that you feel a stretch in your back leg's hip flexor but not so big that you lose your balance or have to bring your chest forward to avoid falling over.

2. Lower the back knee until it is almost touching the floor. Keep your front foot firmly planted and do not rise onto your toes. Engage your core to keep your torso erect and prevent rounding or softening. Keep the back straight and tall *(b)*.

REPETITION

Complete 10 repetitions, then switch to the right leg. Or, for a greater challenge, you can alternate legs with each repetition.

TIPS

- Make sure the front knee does not extend past the toes.
- Sit the hips and glutes down and back rather than straight down.
- To bring the right foot to the starting position, drive through the front heel to engage the glutes.

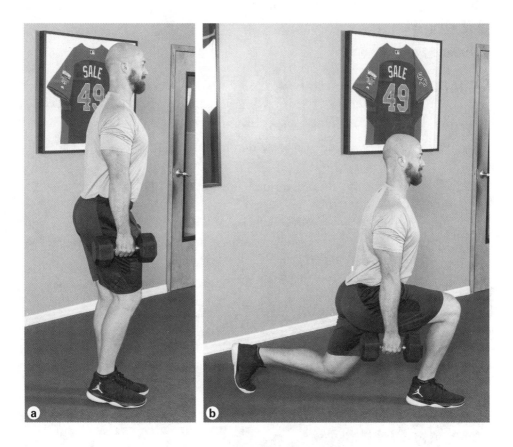

DUMBBELL OVERHEAD PRESS

This exercise teaches the athlete to stabilize with a load overhead. Be sure you are safe and stable when pressing anything overhead. It is important to learn how to stabilize the entire body when lifting weight of any amount overhead. In order to prevent injuries, everything must work together, from the feet being firmly planted into the floor to a strong, straight torso and tight core.

TECHNIQUE

1. Stand with the feet hip-distance apart. Hold a dumbbell in each hand in front of your shoulders, with elbows bent and palms facing forward (a).

2. Extend the arms as you push the dumbbells overhead (b). To create the proper dumbbell path, think about making a triangle with the dumbbells throughout the movement. The three points of the triangle are from the inside head of each dumbbell (the part closest to your shoulders) to the peak at the top where they meet over your head. As the dumbbells rise, keep them in line with your ears; do not let them float forward or extend backward. Keeping them on this path will make the move easier and will reduce the risk of injury.

REPETITION

Complete 10 repetitions.

VARIATION

A push press involves the lower half of the body and assists the lift on the way up. To do the push press, do a "dip-drive."

1. From the start position, slightly bend the knees and dip your backside back a little.

2. As you extend the arms overhead, drive up with the tension in the legs created from the dip.

3. Return to the start position, with the knees slightly bent and backside sitting back. Don't rush the movement and start your dip before the dumbbells have reached their starting position.

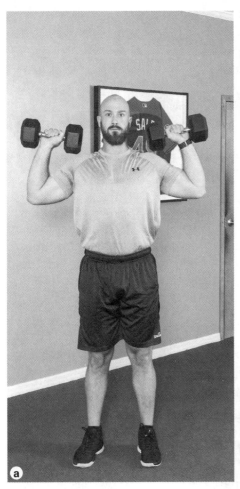 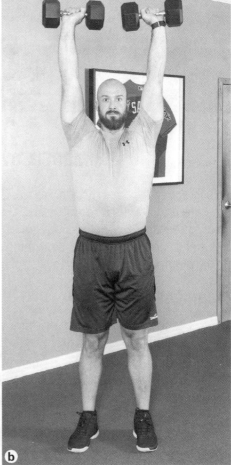

DUMBBELL HIGH PULL

The high pull may be the most complex exercise in the dumbbell group. The high pull is similar to an upright row, but it incorporates triple extension. Triple extension is the extension of the ankle, knee, and hip joints in succession. It is a fast, powerful lift designed to teach explosive, but controlled, movements.

TECHNIQUE

1. Stand with the feet hip-distance part, knees slightly bent, and the torso hinging forward from the hips at about a 45-degree angle. Hold a dumbbell in each hand, arms extended and palms facing the legs so that the dumbbells hang in front of your body just above your knees *(a)*.

2. Explosively extend your hips upward and forward and rise onto your toes as you pull the dumbbells up toward your face, making sure that your elbows stay up and your palms remain facing your body *(b)*. When you reach the highest point of the high pull you will be in full triple extension. This means you have some degree of extension through your back—allowing the path of the dumbbells to stay close to your body, thus making it easier to control the weight—and full extension in your knees and ankles as you lift onto your toes *(c)*.

3. After you have reached your highest point of the high pull, return to the start position in a controlled manner so that the dumbbells don't yank

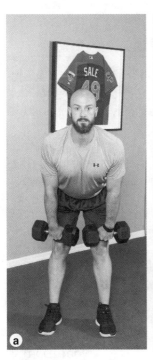
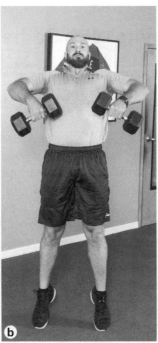
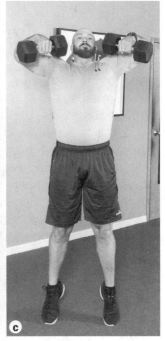

your upper body down with them as they fall. Take a moment to reset before completing the next repetition.

REPETITION
Complete 10 repetitions.

TIPS

- These movements focus on body control; lack of control can lead to sloppy technique and injury.
- All of the power and momentum of this move comes from the hips, not the arms, so remember that when you are completing the high pull, it is not an upright row. Your arms are there only to guide the dumbbells up and down.
- Take your time, make sure your body is properly aligned, and create tension throughout your body to produce the force necessary to move the weight.

_____

As previously mentioned, dumbbells are a great tool for both ongoing training and for teaching an athlete to move in a variety of planes. And if you're working in a small facility or home gym, you can perform all of your weight workouts with dumbbells without compromising your ability to develop greater strength and stability.

Training With Barbells

There is no doubt that you can lift more weight using a barbell than dumbbells. For instance, you may be able to bench 200 pounds (91 kg) for five reps with a bar, but you may be able to bench press only 100 pounds (45 kg) with dumbbells.

Most people are able to lift about 20 percent more weight using a barbell than the combined weight of two dumbbells for the same exercise. This is because they use fewer stabilizing muscles on barbell exercises, which allows them to lift more weight.

Although you can increase your strength, muscle mass, and the amount of weight you lift with both barbells and dumbbells, it is often easier to do so with barbells, especially when you use heavier weights. This is because dumbbell weight increases by 5 pounds (2.3 kg), meaning that the smallest increase in load is 10 pounds (4.5 kg) (5 pounds per dumbbell). In contrast, you can increase the total load of barbells by just 5 pounds (a 2.5-pound [1 kg] plate on each side), which can make it easier to steadily progress and build more muscle and strength over time.

One of the biggest components of our training in the weight room is teaching athletes how to properly execute Olympic lifts. It is as important to our weight training as Pilates is for our core development and overall body

Coaching Tip

When teaching a new exercise, we often begin (especially with young athletes) by teaching the new movement pattern using light dumbbells. Once the athletes understand how their body moves and how to perform the technique correctly, they graduate to a barbell with little or no weight. As their technique improves, they gradually increase the weight on the bar.

awareness and flexibility. As it is with dumbbells, it is also crucial to use barbells safely and with a spotter, especially as you're challenging yourself or your athletes with heavier weights and more complex exercises.

Barbells are at the core of most strength and conditioning programs. They assist in creating the strength and power that is needed for speed. Remember, it is impossible to develop speed in a weak athlete who is unable to create power. Barbell exercises are an effective way to develop strength and in turn increase speed.

Fundamental Olympic Lifts

Olympic weightlifting is based on two exercises: the snatch and the clean and jerk. These two exercises force an athlete's body into positions that require them not only to create force, but also to absorb it. Think about the ramifications behind that sentence. If you're a power forward for your basketball team, your effectiveness is based on how much force you can create (jumping) and how well you absorb the external bumping around you. These two lifts, which teach athletes to produce force and absorb impact, beautifully relate to most sports. Olympic weightlifting, if taught correctly, may just be the best tool for preparing athletes for the field or court.

Olympic Weightlifting

The benefits of Olympic lifting are numerous when taught in a safe, progressive manner. To perform these lifts efficiently, you must possess a strong posterior chain—the biceps femoris, gluteus maximus, erector spinae, trapezius, and posterior deltoids—which allows for safe functional patterns.

The posterior chain should be addressed first without a significant load. The Pilates and med ball exercises described in previous chapters will prepare the body for heavier loads. Once the chain is established, Olympic lifting is an excellent way to address propulsion and absorption.

It is essential in both these lifts that you explode off the ground in a controlled manner. The force production that these lifts demand translates wonderfully to the field or court. Some coaches may not emphasize the importance of correctly absorbing the bar. During the catch phase of the clean, the athletes pull themselves under the bar and stabilize it once their feet meet the ground. Unless the athlete is lifting at high percentages, I like to see them absorb the bar when they meet it. (By high percentages, we mean the percent of an athlete's one repetition maximum [1RM]. If the heaviest load is 100 pounds and that is the athlete's 1RM, and the athlete is working at 70 percent, then that is the athlete's high percent.). This means that they don't fall directly into their front squat during the catch phase. The athlete must stabilize the load and learn to absorb the external factors. Imagine the usefulness to an athlete. Not only do the lifts train for power, but they also teach the athlete how to absorb force.

Let's take football as an example. The most important skills for a running back are creating force and preparing his body to take hits. The power clean develops these skills. The force application through the floor and how the

Rick's Tips

I was given the opportunity to learn Olympic lifts from two of the best coaches in the country, Al Vermeil and Dragomir Cioroslan.

Al Vermeil is the only strength coach to have world championship rings from both the National Football League and the National Basketball Association. He is also the only strength coach who has worked in the NFL, NBA, and Major League Baseball. I was fortunate enough to train under him while he was with the Chicago Bulls.

Dragomir Cioroslan is the director of international strategies and development for the United States Olympic Committee. He was the USA Weightlifting coach for 13 years. In 2006, he became the director of International Strategies and Development at the United States Olympic Committee.

When Al gave me an opportunity to intern with the Chicago Bulls, he gave me a career. He taught me how to prepare athletes to perform Olympic lifts and start them with proper progressions. That position turned into an opportunity for me to finish school in Colorado Springs and work directly under Dragomir at the U.S. Olympic Training Center (OTC) where he was the head coach of USA Weightlifting. I couldn't have asked for a better environment in which to learn.

At the OTC, my job was to calculate the intensity and volume of the percentages and reps lifted throughout the week for Super Squad 2000 (the Olympic hopefuls). I also assisted in training the junior squad for USA Weightlifting. For two years, I spent four hours a day in the weight room coaching and learning from other coaches. It was some of the best coaching I have ever seen and it was incredible! It taught me how to refine athlete progression during each training phase, and that Olympic lifting is just as neurologically draining as it is physically. Last and definitely not least, the experience engrained in me the proper ways to teach and implement a jerk, snatch, and clean. So much so, that when on the platform in my own gym, I feel a certain peace come over me. Al has been essential to that comfort with training. To this day, he still pushes the envelope in the strength and conditioning field, and constantly searches for knowledge. That's why he's the best. I know if I follow that hunger, I will do right by my athletes and give them the best coaching I'm capable of.

athlete meets the bar directly correlate to the field of play. It's a lift that demands power.

A negative side of Olympic lifting is that it is often taught incorrectly. Either the athlete isn't ready for demanding lifts, or the coach can't put together proper progressions to teach the lifts effectively. One method we use to help coaches in this area is summed up in this statement: If you haven't felt it, you can't teach it. Not only do our coaches hold degrees in human performance, but they also spend many hours as our interns or apprentices before working with our clients. They undergo extensive training in all areas of the Olympic lifts before teaching them, and they have all performed these lifts thousands of time and can execute them perfectly. Olympic lifts should be repeated no more than three times. These are not exercises that are repeated in multiple sets or repetitions as other strength exercises may be.

HIGH PULL

As discussed earlier with the dumbbell high pull, a barbell high pull is a great way to learn bar path and speed. It's the first step to mastering Olympic-style lifting. It teaches an athlete where the bar is located in space and time, and encourages the proper extension of the spine needed to perform the clean and snatch properly. The high pull is similar to an upright row, but it incorporates triple extension. Triple extension is the extension of the ankle, knee, and hip joints in succession that allows moves to be explosive and powerful.

TECHNIQUE

1. To start the high pull, get into the hang position, with the barbell hanging in front of your body just above the knees *(a)*.

2. Before you release out of your hang position into triple extension, create tension throughout your posterior chain and arms to create a whip effect on the bar.

3. From the hang position, explosively extend your hips upward and forward so that your back is in extension. Leading with your elbows, pull the bar up toward your face. Your elbows stay up and do not fall backward so that your wrists turn over and your palms face out *(b)*.

4. When you reach the highest point of the exercise, you should be in full triple extension. You have some degree of extension through your back— which allows the bar path to stay close to your body, making it easier to control the weight—and full extension in your knees and ankles, and you are on your toes *(c)*.

5. The power and momentum of this move comes from the hips, not the arms, like in an upright row. Your arms are there only to guide the bar up and down.

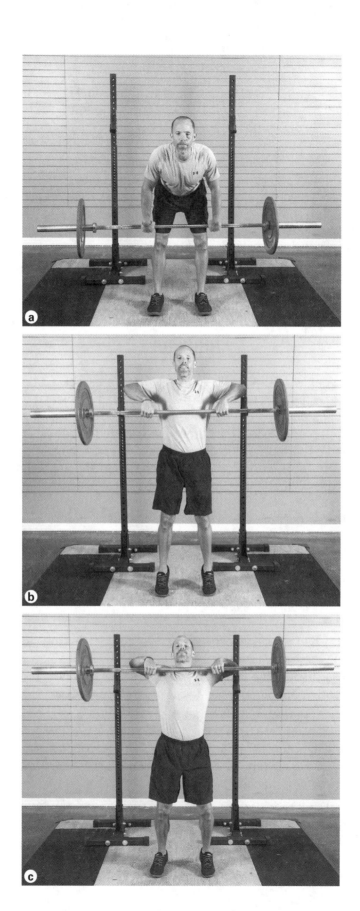

6. After you have reached the highest point of the exercise, let the bar fall in a controlled manner so that it doesn't yank the upper body down as the bar falls.

REPETITION

Repeat three times. Once the bar has come back to the original starting position, take a second to reset your hang position and then repeat the exercise as necessary.

TIPS

- These movements focus on body control. Lack of control can lead to sloppy technique or injury depending on the external load.
- Don't rush through this move by jumping right back into your hang position after the bar comes back down. Take your time, and make sure your body is properly aligned and you have tension throughout to create the force necessary to move the weight.

HANG CLEAN

The hang clean develops impulse: reaction time based on neurological response instead of being cued each time. In the hang position, you don't have a lot of time to create force, so you must create even more speed neurologically and physically. When performing the clean, start from the hang positon. This teaches bar path and bar speed and meeting the bar in the catch. Depending on the requirements of the sport, some athletes will progress to the power clean, which has a lower starting position. Athletes should learn to create force in the body position they use in their particular sport. For example, a second baseman has no reason to change this start position. But a catcher would progress to the ground and the power clean because the athlete must generate force from a low position. On a football team, the lineman would do power cleans from the floor and the skill position players start from the hang. Training should be position specific and targeted to the athlete and the requirements of their sport. The clean can start from the hang position, mid-shin, or from the floor. One of the keys to Olympic lifting is that during the pull, you jump to create the force to drive the weight up explosively.

TECHNIQUE

1. Stand with the feet hip-distance apart, torso hinged forward from the hips at about a 45-degree angle, and the barbell hanging in front of your body just above the knees. The grip for the clean is just wider than shoulder width on the bar, palms facing you *(a)*. A grip that is too narrow or too wide causes problems once you get to the catch position.

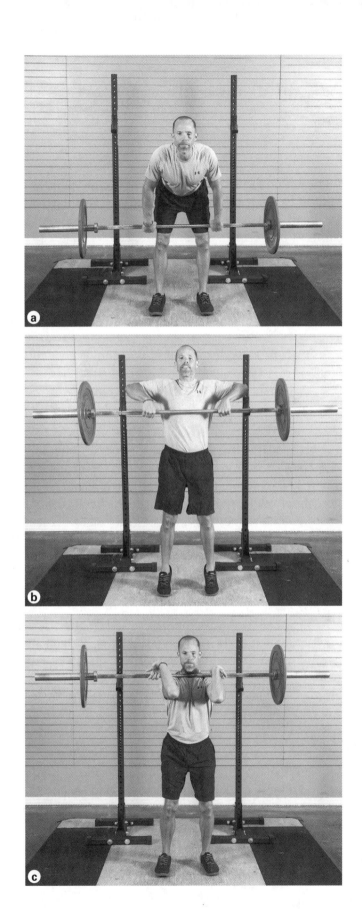

2. Just as you would with the high pull, explosively extend your hips upward and forward so that your back is in extension. As you pull, jump while the bar is coming up to help create force and whip on the bar. Leading with your elbows, pull the bar up toward your face, keeping your elbows up until you have reached the top of the pull *(b)*.

3. At the high point in the pull, punch your elbows down and under the bar, finishing with your palms facing up.

4. Catch the bar by making a shelf across your clavicles. Keep a slight bend in your knees to help absorb the force from the weight and bar *(c)*. The more weight on the bar, the lower your catch position. It is important that when you enter your catch position, you hold your elbows up as high as possible. Allowing the elbows to drop may lead to a poor catch position, a failed clean, or potential injury.

5. After you catch the bar, stand up tall while keeping your elbows up and hold the finished position before returning to the start position.

REPETITION

Repeat three times.

SNATCH

The snatch is one of the fastest ways to create extension. Many of our skill players execute this lift. It is an easier exercise to learn than the clean, but it requires more bar speed. It is perfect for an infielder, point guard, or wide receiver because the force application has to be strong and it engrains the movements of the fast-twitch muscles. The athlete can transfer the skill onto the field quickly.

TECHNIQUE

1. The snatch uses a wider grip than the clean. A good gauge for grip width is to position your hands so that the bar hangs at the height of your pubic bone. Stand with the feet hip-distance apart. Hinge the torso forward from the hips to about a 45-degree angle, with the bar hanging above the knees *(a)*.

2. Leading with the elbows, pull the bar toward you as in a high pull. As you pull, explode up from the feet to create a whip effect on the bar *(b)*.

3. Once the bar has reached the high point of the high pull, flip your wrists over so that your palms face away from you.

4. Extend your arms to push the bar overhead as you pull your body under the bar into a semisquat position *(c)*. This position allows for better control and absorption from the bar.

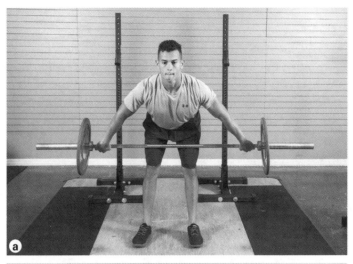

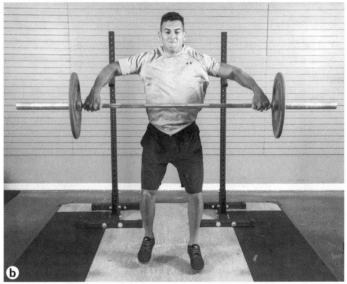

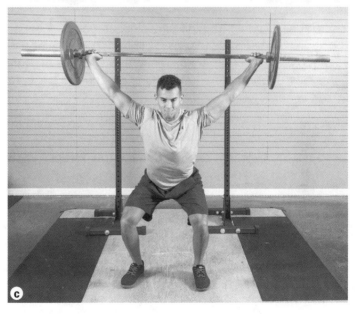

5. Lock your arms out once the bar has reached its peak, and extend the legs to stand up tall with the bar to complete the snatch.

REPETITION

Repeat three times.

JERK AND PUSH PRESS

Overhead movements from a standing position provide more effective training than exercises such as the bench press. Why? Because they require coordination and stabilization of the entire body as the bar is lifted overhead. The bench press is performed in a supine position, and not many sports are played while lying on your back.

TECHNIQUE

1. Stand with the feet hip-distance apart, and hold the barbell with a pronated grip. The bar rests across your clavicles and upper chest *(a)*.
2. Sit your backside down and back into a semisquat position. This will allow you to use your lower half during the push and achieve triple extension.
3. Push through the ground and drive the bar up off your shoulders to an extended overhead position.
4. As you reach the top of the push, lock your arms out with the bar slightly behind your head to allow for greater stabilization as you stick the press *(b)*.
5. Return the bar to your chest.

REPETITION

Repeat three times.

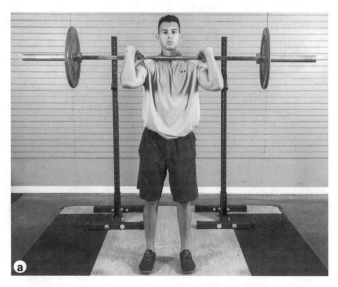

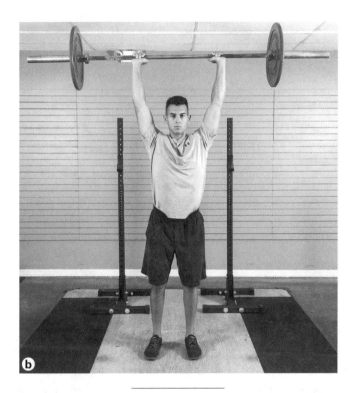

Barbell and dumbbell movements are important components of an athlete's training program. They should serve as one modality that fits into a comprehensive approach that meets the athlete's needs, and the sole method for building strength and power. I often see coaches fixate on these Olympic lifting movements, but they need to understand they're not training an Olympic lifter. They're training an athlete who plays a game that is outside the weight room.

Now that you understand the benefits of each method of strength training, how do you choose between them? Start by determining what your athlete needs. What are their strengths and weaknesses? Constantly assess an athlete's development and progress. Are dumbbells or barbells better for a particular exercise? What about resistance bands? There is no one way to reach an athlete's goals. Be vigilant in assessing whether the program you have designed uses the best strategy for the athlete for a particular training session.

Next Steps

In chapter 8, we will introduce several programs for movement preparation, recovery, and everything in between. These programs will help you establish the right training session at the right time as your level of competency increases.

PART III | THE WORKOUTS

8 | **Foundational Workouts**

You have been given a huge amount of information over the past seven chapters, and it can be overwhelming trying to determine where to begin. The first step is to create your foundation. Think in terms of architecture. A structurally sound building starts with a strong foundation. If there are cracks in your foundation, nothing will align correctly.

The workouts in this chapter serve a variety of uses. Perhaps you are already fit, and you want to use everything we have shared to improve your overall performance level. Maybe you are just coming out of rehab after surgery. If so, these workouts will help you address deficiencies and build strength where you need it. And if you are just beginning a new fitness regimen, congratulations! The workouts will give you a solid base from which to develop fitness, strength, and flexibility.

This chapter outlines programs that incorporate preparation moves and exercises that include myofascial release, joint articulation, glute activation, dynamic warm-up, Pilates, and medicine ball and resistance band training. These programs are ideal for preparing your body for additional training on the same day, developing a strong and flexible base, and providing the recovery that will prepare you for the advanced programs in chapter 9.

Every day you wake up with a new body. Energy levels vary, workouts and sports may make you sore, sleep patterns may change, and nutrition may differ from one day to the next. You do not need to repeat the same program every day. It's OK to vary them from day to day. However, selecting the correct program depends on where you are in your training cycle as well as the other factors just listed. You may find it beneficial to continue with the fundamental programs in chapters 8 and 9 for the first month of your development. You will notice that we repeat many of the

We use the workouts in this book with our clients and incorporate the techniques we have shared with you into our personal programs as well. To achieve the best results, it's important to understand the process and then follow through. We cannot increase the capacity of our workouts and challenge our bodies in new ways without having a strong, flexible foundation and the knowledge needed to develop the best recovery programs. You are designing your body for the job you want it to do. Knowing your starting point, structuring your long- and short-term game plan, and training consistently will allow you to reach and possibly exceed your expectations. Remember that being consistent and trusting the process is imperative. Wavering or resisting any part of the work will lead to falling short of your goals.

beginning prep movements throughout each of our programs. You will incorporate a variety of movement patterns every time you work out in order to prepare your body correctly for the training that will follow.

Our athletes perform similar warm-up exercises before starting their workout for the day. These patterns may include the foam roller, the articulation series, Pilates, and of course their dynamic warm-up before they ever touch a piece of equipment that day. The length of their workout may exceed the standard one-hour training session in order for them to warm up, work out, and stretch afterward.

You Know Your Body Better Than Anyone

As we mentioned earlier, it's important to select a workout space that is safe, well equipped, and conducive to your training for the day. But in addition to your environment and variations in how you feel from one day to the next, you also need to take your overall physical and mental health into consideration. Are you having a stressful week? Is your body tired from overtraining? Are you finding it hard to get your motor running today? These are all things to keep in mind when selecting your daily workout. Sometimes we need a push. We need to feel our endorphins kicking in and our heart pumping to get us into a better mood or back on track. Other days we need to take things a bit more slowly, such as after a huge race or being sick. Remember that you are in charge. You know your body better than anyone. Challenge yourself. You're reading this book in order to challenge yourself and improve your overall performance.

If you are dealing with medical issues, injuries (new or old), surgeries, emotional issues, and so on, you must take them into account when selecting your workout for the day, week, and month. If your doctor or physical therapist has given you limitations, by all means follow them. We know that athletes like to push themselves harder than most. But trust us, there is a limit to the "no pain, no gain" theory. Pain as in muscle soreness from an intense training session is quite different from injury pain or joint pain. Listen to your body. Know your limitations. And above all, be smart about your workout selections. You can always make things more challenging once you have created a strong foundation. Nothing good comes from pushing your body too hard too quickly and developing an injury.

Selecting Workout Programs

After reading chapters 1 through 7, you have gained insight into the Beyond Motion philosophy and the movement patterns needed to become a stronger, faster, better equipped athlete. Now it's time to put these exercises into action and train. Knowing what to do and when to do it is a science. Yes, programming and training should be approached with a technician's mind-set. Going to the gym to lift just for the sake of getting in a workout doesn't create a better athlete. Planning, programming, execution, and persistence do.

Unfortunately, there is no one-size-fits-all answer to the programming question. Not everyone should follow the same program at the same time for the same length of time. So, you, and not us, need to answer the question of what your body needs to do for your workout. Use the primary assessment in chapter 2 to determine a solid starting point.

We are working under the assumption that not only have you already taken your primary assessment, but that you have read the goal-setting and game plan information in chapter 2 as well. We know that by following the goal-setting exercises, you will gain a strong understanding of why you are training this way and the benefits that you will gain by following the programs.

The frequency and duration of the workouts differ from person to person depending on what the rest of the training week, games, and field or court time may entail. What we can share with you is that your warm-up alone should take at least 20 minutes. Your warm-up should include your roller work, joint articulation series if needed, Pilates, and at least part, if not the entire, dynamic warm-up series. These movements prepare your body to train. If you're brand new to this type of training, following the entire foam roller, joint articulation, Pilates, and dynamic warm-up series could be your entire workout for the day. For others, this provides just a warm-up.

Even though your programming will advance and you will select new workouts to help you reach your goals, you will always begin with a warm-up. And, when you find a warm-up that works for you, you could follow the same protocol each time. Before every workout, Rick does the same warm-up. This includes foam roller, joint articulation, glute activation, and dyno. Only after that is his body ready to begin training.

Program 1: Warm Up Your Nervous System

Energizing and engaging your body for movement is the ideal prepping point and should be completed before every workout. The first two programs may be used interchangeably, depending on how your body feels that day and the actual workout that follows. Some days you may feel lethargic or groggy and program 1 may wake you up. On other days, tightness may be your main concern, and program 2 may be a better choice. Just make sure to use one of the initial warm-up programs before each of your workouts. Do not go straight into any of the additional programs without taking the time to prepare your body.

Warm-Up

Modality	Exercise	Page
Foam roller	Nervous system activation	40
Foam roller	Head tilt	41
Foam roller	Head nod	42
Foam roller	Chest opener	43
Foam roller	Supine back roll	48
Foam roller	Hamstring stretch	50
Foam roller	Quadriceps release	53
Foam roller	IT band release	52
Foam roller	Toe tap	57
Foam roller	Side stretch with low lunge	46
Joint articulation series	Start with feet, working upward as needed.	66

Program 2: Stretch Out

This program is ideal for days when you feel like your hips and hamstrings are too tight. For some people that may be a daily occurrence, and for others it occurs occasionally depending on the workouts and activities completed the day before. Regardless of which category you fall into, the following exercises will allow you to feel more open and able to move with greater freedom and ease. This chapter should be used for warm-ups or by those who are brand new to these types of exercises, need foundation workouts, or are postrehabilitation. The exercises should be used prior to adding additional weight-based workouts and by people who are looking for a great Pilates workout.

Stretch Out

Modality	Exercise	Page
Foam roller	Supine back roll	48
Foam roller	Glute release	49
Foam roller	Quadriceps release	53
Foam roller	IT band release	52
Foam roller	Hamstring stretch	50
Joint articulation series	Ankle series	66
Joint articulation series	Knee circle	68
Joint articulation series	Hip series Reevaluate after each section of the joint articulation series to determine whether you need to continue past your hips and complete the entire joint articulation series.	69
Pilates	Spine stretch forward	102
Pilates	Saw	122
Pilates	Spine twist	120
Foam roller	Swan	61
Pilates	Swimming	131
Pilates	Side-lying clam	128
Foam roller	Side stretch with low lunge	46

Program 3: Pilates Get to the Core of It

When you strengthen your powerhouse, you improve your overall performance level. This warm-up engages your entire powerhouse, working every part of your core.

Pilates for the Core

Modality	Exercise	Page
Pilates	Quadruped bird dog	104
Pilates	Chest lift	110
Pilates	Hundreds	111
Pilates	Single-leg stretch	113
Pilates	Double-leg stretch	114
Pilates	Crisscross oblique	115
Pilates	Hamstring pull	116
Pilates	Teaser prep	143
Pilates	Roll-up	118
Pilates	Pilates push-up	146
Pilates	Leg pull front	142
Pilates	Swimming	131
Pilates	Rolling like a ball	134
Pilates	Standing roll-down	147

Program 4: Loosen Your Tight Back

By increasing flexibility throughout your posterior chain, your movement patterns and agility will improve tenfold.

Loosen Up

Modality	Exercise	Page
Foam roller	Supine back roll	48
Foam roller	Glute release	49
Foam roller	Hamstring stretch	50
Foam roller	IT band release	52
Foam roller	Quadriceps release	53
Pilates	Bridge	107
Pilates	Spine stretch forward	102
Pilates	Spine twist	120
Pilates	Saw	122
Pilates	Hundreds	111
Pilates	Hamstring pull	116
Pilates	Roll-up	118
Pilates	Mermaid	138
Foam roller	Shoulder shrug	60
Foam roller	Swan	61
Joint articulation series	Follow through from ankles upward as needed.	66

Program 5: Getting Your Glutes to Fire

Think of your glutes as your power zone and your shock absorbers. They must work correctly for you to become an effective mover; there is no way around it.

Glute Exercises

Modality	Exercise	Page
Foam roller	Glute release	49
Foam roller	Quadriceps release	53
Foam roller	IT band release	52
Foam roller	Hamstring stretch	50
Foam roller	Calf stretch	51
Foam roller	Supine back roll	48
Joint articulation series	Complete series as needed with repeat check-ins.	66
Dynamic warm-up	Full sequence	73
Glute activation series	Full series	86
Pilates	Side-lying clam	128
Pilates	Lift and lower	125

Program 6: Strengthen Your Powerhouse

Your powerhouse includes the muscles from your pelvic floor to your diaphragm in the front of your body, and from your pelvic floor through your middle thoracic spine on the back of your body. Stabilizing and strengthening this area allows for greater power, strength, and range of motion.

Powerhouse

Modality	Exercise	Page
Foam roller	Supine back roll	48
Foam roller	Glute release	49
Foam roller	Hamstring stretch	50
Foam roller	IT band release	52
Foam roller	Quadriceps release	53
Pilates	Bridge	107
Pilates	Hundreds	111
Pilates	Single-leg stretch	113
Pilates	Double-leg stretch	114
Pilates	Crisscross oblique	115
Pilates	Hamstring pull	116
Pilates	Roll-up	118
Pilates	Spine twist	120
Pilates	Saw	122
Pilates	Swan	129
Pilates	Swimming	131
Pilates	Mermaid	138
Pilates	Rollover	139
Pilates	Teaser prep or full teaser	143 or 144
Resistance band	Reverse fly	187
Resistance band	Seated row	190

Pilates Workouts

Basic Pilates Workout

Modality	Exercise	Page
Pilates	Spine stretch forward	102
Pilates	Pelvic curl	106
Pilates	Bridge	107
Pilates	Circle	126
Pilates	Chest lift	110
Pilates	Hundreds	111
Pilates	Saw	122
Pilates	Spine twist	120
Pilates	Side-kick series	123
Pilates	Leg pull front	142
Pilates	Swimming	131
Pilates	Rolling like a ball	134
Pilates	Mermaid	138
Pilates	Pilates push-up	146
Pilates	Roll-up	118

Intermediate Pilates Workout

Modality	Exercise	Page
Pilates	Pelvic curl	106
Pilates	Bridge	107
Pilates	Chest lift	110
Pilates	Hundreds	111
Pilates	Hamstring pull	116
Pilates	Single-leg stretch	113
Pilates	Double-leg stretch	114
Pilates	Crisscross oblique	115
Pilates	Saw	122
Pilates	Roll-up	118
Pilates	Spine twist	120
Pilates	Shoulder bridge	108
Pilates	Rolling like a ball	134
Pilates	Side-kick series	123
Pilates	Swan	129
Pilates	Swimming	131
Pilates	Spine stretch forward	102
Pilates	Pilates push-up	146
Pilates	Leg pull front	142
Pilates	Standing roll-down	147

Full-Body Workout

Full-Body Workout

Modality	Exercise	Page
Foam roller	IT band release	52
Foam roller	Quadriceps release	53
Joint articulation series	Toes up	66
Joint articulation series	Toes down	67
Dynamic warm-up	Full sequence	73
Glute activation series	Lateral glute walk	87
Pilates	Hundreds	111
Pilates	Hamstring pull	116
Pilates	Crisscross oblique	115
Pilates	Quadruped bird dog	104
Pilates	Roll-up	118
Pilates	Leg pull	136
Medicine ball	Hammer throw	161
Resistance band	Squat	178
Dumbbell	Dumbbell overhead press	201
Dumbbell	Dumbbell row	199
Pilates	Mermaid	138

Amy's Story

In 2016, I decided to challenge myself by doing something completely out of my comfort zone, so I trained and competed in a figure competition (physique exhibition event; think in terms of bodybuilding just not as muscular) in 2017. I have spent most of my life working out, but training with this kind of specificity was something completely new for me. While I had many months to prepare, I wanted to make sure that I was spending my time wisely and incorporating everything I knew about weight training and Pilates to create efficient and effective workouts. I spent time analyzing my body and injuries, movement patterns, nutritional concerns, and what I needed to accomplish to succeed at the contest. I set my goals using the goal-setting techniques we shared with you in chapter 2, so that every day I was able to maximize my time and my energy. I prepared my body for each workout with the joint articulation series and foam roller.

Typical body-building workouts are organized into splits in which particular muscle groups are worked at certain times, for example legs and glutes one day and upper body the next. And while this is helpful for achieving your overall goal, it's not the only way to train. I wanted to not only look symmetrical, but I also wanted to make sure that as I increased my training, my body functioned well and didn't become too tired and damaged from the increased training volume. My training program varied from week to week and month to month. As my strength increased and my body fat decreased, it became even more important for me to maintain my Pilates practice to ensure that I was maintaining my core strength, flexibility, and all of the muscle definition I knew the judges would look for. All of my Pilates sessions are complete, whole body workouts and were the ideal balance for all of the additional weight workouts and cardio sessions I completed each day.

While about 75 percent of my Pilates workouts included Pilates equipment, I always incorporated some of the mat exercises into my program. The moves became the glue that held everything together. And the hard work and correct programming paid off. At my first competition in November 2017, I won first place in the following categories: Figure Debut (first time on stage), Figure Masters (women over 35), Figure Open (women of every age and every height), and second place in Bikini Open. I was also fortunate enough to earn my pro card for Figure Open.

As I prepared for my next contest the following summer, I continued to increase my Pilates workouts to match my training. Some days I did Pilates and cardio, other days I added Pilates into my training session, and at other times I did Pilates early in the day and trained with weights in the afternoon or evening. Again, the patterns worked. The second contest was much larger and the competition was tough. I placed second in one category and third in another.

Being just a few weeks away from my upcoming figure competition, I can tell you that I am working even harder to expound upon my Pilates practice.

As I continue to lift heavier weights and challenge my body to do more, I know it is even more important to maintain this portion of my training.

While I change my Pilates workouts to counterbalance whatever other workout I may have done that day, the series of five including hamstring pull are some of my go-to exercises. The side-kick series is great for sculpting your glutes and the prone series, including swimming and swan, is excellent for developing the posterior chain. I love how Pilates builds my endurance and warms me up for whatever else I want to include. Quadruped is a great exercise to restabilize my body and get an amazing cross-body connection. Leg pull opens my chest and shoulders while working my core, especially after a heavy lift. Each exercise offers so many benefits that I can spend days creating a variety of workouts lasting from 10 to 60 minutes and never get bored. Partnering Pilates exercises with everything else we have taught you in this book allows for endless possibilities.

If you're looking to add a more advanced Pilates workout to your program, try these exercises and see what they do for you.

Figure Prep Intermediate Pilates Workout

Modality	Exercise Name	Page
Pilates	Pelvic curl	106
Pilates	Bridge	107
Pilates	Shoulder bridge	108
Pilates	Chest lift	110
Pilates	Hundreds	111
Pilates	Single-leg stretch	113
Pilates	Hamstring pull	116
Pilates	Roll-up	118
Pilates	Saw	122
Pilates	Pilates push-up	146
Pilates	Swimming	131
Pilates	Single-leg kick	132
Pilates	Rolling like a ball	134
Pilates	Upper and lower lift	127
Pilates	Side-lying clam	128
Pilates	Leg pull	136
Pilates	Teaser	144
Pilates	Mermaid	138
Pilates	Quadruped bird dog	104
Pilates	Standing roll-down	147

Next Steps

After working for a few weeks with the programs we have outlined, you should notice quite an improvement in how your body looks, feels, and performs. For some of you, these programs will be your mainstay and you will continue working with them for the next few months. For others of you, it's time to up your level of intensity and move on to more specific program options in chapter 9.

The programs in chapter 9 address specific sports and goals. Whether you play tennis, pickleball, golf, baseball, or volleyball or compete in triathlons, we have you covered. While each program is designed to meet a goal such as developing overall fitness or power or to benefit a specific sport, we know that not every workout is suitable for everybody. Peruse the programs to find one that suits you best at the time. You can always revisit other workouts and add them to your program later.

9 | Intermediate, Advanced, and Sport-Specific Workouts

Chapter 8 taught you the basics of the workouts and prepared you for what comes next. Once you have been working with the fundamental programs in chapter 8 for your first four to six weeks, it may be time to increase your training in order to develop an even greater strength base.

Now the real work begins as you prepare for what you love to do most. Regardless of whether you are a recreational, amateur, or professional athlete, having a coach behind you is important. Perhaps you are fortunate enough to have access to your coach or trainer 24 hours a day. But for most people that is not possible, which is why we created this book. Use this chapter to take your training to the next level. You will be able to select and implement a variety of programs that will help you become a well-rounded athlete.

Chapter 9 offers general workouts you can use no matter what sport or activity you participate in, along with workouts designed for specific sports. We use these workouts with our clients every day. Remember, your workout program should be based not only on the goals you established in chapter 2, but also on where your body and training are right now. Of course, not every workout is suitable for every person. You know your body and what you can tolerate at any given moment. If one day you feel amazing and super strong, push yourself a bit further. If, on the other hand, yesterday's workout has you feeling tired and sore, maybe today should be a recovery day. You can continue using the programs in chapter 8 as needed as well. Many of those programs are perfect for recovery days.

Programming is a science and an art all in one. Every athlete we work with has an individual program created weekly that progresses from the previous week. A good coach may sense a lack of energy in an athlete or poor body language on a particular day. This is when they evaluate the situation and go ahead with what they had planned or pivot and adjust the program so that it fits the athlete's current needs. A good program is like a good game plan. Not everything will go your way, so you have to be ready to pivot and make adjustments when needed.

If you are a coach using these workouts with your athletes, be smart about it. If you're coaching an individual, develop workouts that minimize their deficiencies and fine-tune their strengths. If you're coaching a team, you might customize workouts based on position or by levels and abilities.

Full-Body Beginner Workout

This workout creates stability within the athlete by addressing the joints and activating the glutes in a sequential manner. This is a great workout for a young athlete who is trying to gain a solid foundation.

Full-Body Beginner Workout

Modality	Exercise	Page
Foam roller	Supine back roll	48
Foam roller	Chest opener	43
Joint articulation series	Ankle series	66
Dynamic warm-up	Walking hamstring	82
Dynamic warm-up	Walking quad	83
Glute activation series	Lateral toe tap	91
Pilates	Pelvic curl	106
Pilates	Bridge	107
Pilates	Hundreds	111
Pilates	Toe tap	103
Pilates	Side-kick series	123
Pilates	Side-lying clam	128
Pilates	Upper and lower lift	127
Pilates	Circle	126
Pilates	Quadruped bird dog	104
Medicine ball	Squat	162
Medicine ball	Wood chop	160
Resistance band	Split squat	179
Resistance band	Squat	178

Full-Body Advanced Beginner Workout

The following workout uses more complex movements and begins to demand more from the athlete's body.

Full-Body Advanced Beginner Workout

Modality	Exercise	Page
Foam roller	Head tilt	41
Foam roller	Head nod	42
Foam roller	Chest opener	43
Joint articulation series	Hip flexion and extension	69
Dynamic warm-up	Walking quad	83
Dynamic warm-up	Walking hamstring	82
Glute activation series	Lateral toe tap	91
Pilates	Quadruped bird dog	104
Pilates	Spine twist	120
Pilates	Hundreds	111
Pilates	Single-leg stretch	113
Pilates	Hamstring pull	116
Pilates	Bridge	107
Pilates	Leg pull front	142
Medicine ball	Wood chop	160
Medicine ball	Diagonal	169
Resistance band	Split squat	179
Glute activation series	Lateral toe taps with band	91
Glute activation series	Lateral glide with band	88

Power Development: Intermediate Workout

In this program the athlete learns to create force while also establishing more core strength.

Power Development: Intermediate Workout

Modality	Exercise	Page
Foam roller	Calf stretch	51
Foam roller	Quadriceps release	53
Joint articulation series	Ankle series	66
Dynamic warm-up	Jumping jack skip	77
Dynamic warm-up	Butt kick	83
Glute activation series	Lateral glide	88
Pilates	Hundreds	111
Pilates	Double-leg stretch	114
Pilates	Neck pull	119
Pilates	Teaser	144
Pilates	Saw	122
Pilates	Rollover	139
Pilates	Double-leg kick	133
Pilates	Rolling like a ball	134
Medicine ball	Overhead slam	166
Olympic lifts	Hang clean	209
Dumbbell	Dumbbell squat	196
Dumbbell	Dumbbell RDL	198

Strength Development: Intermediate Workout

This is a great workout for developing strength. Although it doesn't use a barbell, it is still demanding. The use of dumbbells develops proprioception—the ability to sense the position of the limbs—and recruits the use of stabilizing muscles.

Strength Development: Intermediate Workout

Modality	Exercise	Page
Foam roller	Quadriceps release	53
Foam roller	IT band release	52
Dynamic warm-up	Walking quad	83
Dynamic warm-up	Walking hamstring	82
Glute activation series	Lateral glute walk	87
Pilates	Standing roll-down	147
Pilates	Pilates push-up	146
Pilates	Quadruped bird dog	104
Pilates	Single-leg kick	132
Pilates	Side-kick series: • Front and back kick • Lift and lower • Upper and lower lift • Side-lying clam	123
Pilates	Neck pull	119
Pilates	Crisscross oblique	115
Medicine ball	Wood chop	160
Resistance band	Split squat	179
Dumbbell	Dumbbell squat	196
Dumbbell	Dumbbell RDL	198
Dumbbell	Dumbbell row	199

Rotational Sports (Pickleball, Tennis, Golf)

When we think about rotational sports, we think about mobility and flexibility. Pickleball, tennis, and golf share similar movements and require the same types of flexibility.

Pickleball

This workout is loaded with movements that create a fluid mover.

Pickleball Workout

Modality	Exercise	Page
Foam roller	Chest opener	43
Foam roller	Hamstring stretch	50
Foam roller	Side stretch with low lunge	46
Joint articulation series	Hip flexion and extension	69
Dynamic warm-up	Wide skip	78
Dynamic warm-up	Backward skip with rotation	79
Dynamic warm-up	Lateral skip with rotation	81
Glute activation series	Lateral glute walk	87
Pilates	Spine twist	120
Pilates	Saw	122
Pilates	Hamstring pull	116
Pilates	Swan	129
Pilates	Swimming	131
Pilates	Quadruped bird dog	104
Medicine ball	Hammer throw	161
Medicine ball	Rotational throw	167
Resistance band	Seated row	190

Tennis

This workout develops a more balanced tennis player through strength, med ball, and Pilates exercises.

Tennis Workout

Modality	Exercise	Page
Dynamic warm-up	Relaxed skip series	75
Dynamic warm-up	Wide skip	78
Dynamic warm-up	Lateral skip	80
Dynamic warm-up	Walking hamstring	82
Glute activation series	Lateral glide	88
Glute activation series	Backward 45-degree walk	90
Pilates	Crisscross oblique	115
Pilates	Mermaid	138
Pilates	Pilates push-up	146
Pilates	Roll-up	118
Pilates	Side-lying clam	128
Medicine ball	Big circle	159
Medicine ball	Reverse lunge	163
Medicine ball	Forward lunge	164
Dumbbell	Dumbbell high pull	203
Dumbbell	Dumbbell row	199
Dumbbell	Dumbbell overhead press	201
Dumbbell	Dumbbell reverse lunge	200
Pilates	Standing roll-down	147

Golf

Golfing well requires thoracic mobility and the ability to create torque. This program develops both qualities and is a great addition for golfers of all levels.

Golf Workout

Modality	Exercise	Page
Foam roller	Chest opener	43
Foam roller	Quadriceps release	53
Foam roller	IT band release	52
Foam roller	Hamstring stretch	50
Pilates	Mermaid	64
Joint articulation series	Ankle Series	66
Dynamic warm-up	Jumping jack skip	77
Dynamic warm-up	Wide skip	78
Dynamic warm-up	Butt kick	83
Dynamic warm-up	Walking quad	83
Dynamic warm-up	Dynamic hamstring	84
Pilates	Toe tap	103
Pilates	Chest lift	110
Pilates	Hundreds	111
Pilates	Pelvic curl	106
Pilates	Bridge	107
Pilates	Roll-up	118
Pilates	Saw	122
Pilates	Quadruped bird dog	104
Medicine ball	Squat	162
Medicine ball	Reverse lunge	163
Medicine ball	Forward lunge	164
Medicine ball	Rotational throw	167
Medicine ball	Diagonal	169
Medicine ball	Crunch	170
Dynamic warm-up	Relaxed skip series	75

Lacrosse, Field Hockey, and Soccer

Because these are impact sports, the goal is to create a solid foundation from which an athlete can both exert and absorb force. This workout is one of Rick's favorites.

Lacrosse and Field Hockey Workout

Modality	Exercise	Page
Foam roller	Supine back roll	48
Foam roller	Quadriceps release	53
Foam roller	IT band release	52
Foam roller	Hamstring stretch	50
Foam roller	Calf stretch	51
Joint articulation series	Ankle series	66
Joint articulation series	Hip flexion and extension	69
Dynamic warm-up	Jumping jack skip	77
Dynamic warm-up	Wide skip	78
Dynamic warm-up	Backward 45-degree walk	90
Pilates	Chest lift	110
Pilates	Hundreds	111
Pilates	Hamstring pull	116
Pilates	Saw	122
Pilates	Single-leg kick	132
Pilates	Swimming	131
Pilates	Rolling like a ball	134
Olympic lifts	Hang clean	209
Olympic lifts	Snatch	211
Dumbbell	Dumbbell RDL	198
Dumbbell	Dumbbell reverse lunge	200
Medicine ball	Big circle	159
Medicine ball	Diagonal	169
Medicine ball	Crunch	170

Soccer

This soccer program corrects weaknesses in the foundation of the athlete's movement patterns. The exercises slow the movements so athletes are able to address their strength and stability needs.

Soccer Workout

Exercise	Modality	Page
Foam roller	Nervous system activation series	40
Foam roller	Quadriceps release	53
Foam roller	IT band release	52
Foam roller	Supine back roll	48
Foam roller	Calf stretch	51
Dynamic warm-up	Relaxed skip series	75
Dynamic warm-up	Jumping jack skip	77
Dynamic warm-up	Wide skip	78
Medicine ball	Big circle	159
Medicine ball	Reverse lunge	163
Medicine ball	Forward lunge	164
Dumbbell	Dumbbell squat	196
Dumbbell	Dumbbell RDL	198
Dumbbell	Dumbbell row	199
Dumbbell	Dumbbell overhead press	201
Pilates	Shoulder bridge	108
Pilates	Hundreds	111
Pilates	Crisscross oblique	115
Pilates	Neck pull	119
Pilates	Open-leg rocker	135
Pilates	Side-kick series: • Lift and lower • Front and back kick • Side-lying clam	123

Swimming

The swimming workout focuses on Pilates and med ball exercises. We use this great dry-land workout often with our swimmers.

Swimming Workout

Modality	Exercise	Page
Foam roller	Chest opener	43
Foam roller	Supine back roll	48
Foam roller	Glute release	49
Foam roller	Quadriceps release	53
Dynamic warm-up	Relaxed skip series	75
Dynamic warm-up	Lateral skip	80
Dynamic warm-up	Lateral skip with rotation	81
Pilates	Spine stretch forward	102
Pilates	Pelvic curl	106
Pilates	Bridge	107
Pilates	Hundreds	111
Pilates	Crisscross oblique	115
Pilates	Roll-up	118
Pilates	Leg pull	136
Pilates	Upper and lower lift	127
Pilates	Side-lying clam	128
Medicine ball	Big circle	159
Medicine ball	Wood chop	160
Medicine ball	Hammer throw	161
Medicine ball	Reverse lunge	163
Medicine ball	Squat	162
Medicine ball	Diagonal	169
Medicine ball	Side tap	171

Road Sports
(Cycling, Running)

Road sports can be particularly punishing on your lower-body muscles and require cardiovascular stamina. The following exercises help your heart and lungs work just as efficiently as your legs and hips.

Cycling

Cycling is demanding on the cardiovascular system and shortens the hip flexors. This workout elongates the hip flexors and counteracts the kyphotic position (excessive rounding of the upper and middle back) that cycling requires. We're referring to cycling being a cardio workout that also shortens hip flexors. The workout below is meant to open hip flexors and counter balances kyphotic posture that is innate with many cyclists.

Cycling Workout

Modality	Exercise	Page
Foam roller	Chest opener	43
Foam roller	Supine back roll	48
Foam roller	Glute release	49
Foam roller	Quadriceps release	53
Joint articulation series	Ankle series	66
Joint articulation series	Hip flexion and extension	69
Glute activation series	Lateral glute walk	87
Glute activation series	Lateral glide	88
Glute activation series	Forward 45-degree walk	89
Glute activation series	Backward 45-degree walk	90
Resistance band	Split squat	179
Dumbbell	Dumbbell row	199
Dumbbell	Dumbbell RDL	198
Pilates	Spine stretch forward	102
Pilates	Bridge	107
Pilates	Hamstring pull	116
Pilates	Double-leg stretch	114
Pilates	Crisscross oblique	115
Pilates	Swimming	131
Pilates	Rolling like a ball	134
Pilates	Teaser prep or Full teaser	143 or 144
Pilates	Pilates push-up	146
Pilates	Leg pull	136

Running

Great runners need a strong base and glutes that fire consistently. Great runners must develop strength in their lower body, mobile joints that absorb impact, and glutes that fire consistently. The goal of this program is to prepare athletes for the consistent pounding they endure regardless of whether they run short or long distances.

Running Workout

Modality	Exercise	Page
Foam roller	Supine back roll	48
Foam roller	Glute release	49
Foam roller	Hamstring stretch	50
Foam roller	IT band release	52
Glute activation series	Lateral glute walk	87
Glute activation series	Lateral glide	88
Glute activation series	Forward 45-degree walk	89
Glute activation series	Backward 45-degree walk	90
Pilates	Standing roll-down	147
Pilates	Pilates push-up	146
Pilates	Quadruped bird dog	104
Pilates	Swan	129
Medicine ball	Reverse lunge	163
Medicine ball	Squat	162
Medicine ball	Forward lunge	164
Dumbbell	Dumbbell high pull	203
Dumbbell	Dumbbell row	199
Dumbbell	Dumbbell overhead press	201

Vertical Sports
(Volleyball and Basketball)

Vertical Sports require a component that our bodies are naturally integrated towards. The key is teaching the athlete how to control the takeoff and landing that the sports require. We call them the acceleration phase and negative phase of movement. The program below preps players for this very thing. Remember, the athlete who accelerates and decelerates on a dime is the one who will win the competition.

Volleyball

Because volleyball players jump repeatedly during workouts and games, our workouts for them do not use plyometrics. Why would we train athletes using the same pattern? Instead, the goal is to develop force and strength so that jumps are more powerful, crisper, and vertical.

Volleyball Workout

Modality	Exercise	Page
Dynamic warm-up	Relaxed skip series	75
Dynamic warm-up	Both-arms-up skip	76
Dynamic warm-up	Opposite-arm, opposite-leg skip	77
Dynamic warm-up	Jumping jack skip	77
Glute activation series	Lateral glute walk	87
Glute activation series	Lateral glide	88
Pilates	Standing roll-down	147
Pilates	Leg pull front	142
Pilates	Pilates push-up	146
Pilates	Quadruped bird dog	104
Pilates	Swan	129
Pilates	Swimming	131
Pilates	Rolling like a ball	134
Pilates	Hamstring pull	116
Pilates	Crisscross oblique	115
Pilates	Shoulder bridge	108
Pilates	Mermaid	138
Pilates	Side-lying clam	128
Olympic lifts	High pull	207
Olympic lifts	Hang clean	209
Dumbbell	Dumbbell overhead press	201
Dumbbell	Dumbbell squat	196
Foam roller	Quadriceps release	53
Foam roller	Glute release	49
Foam roller	Hamstring stretch	50

Basketball

This basketball program is aggressive. Snatching, because of the speed component behind it, is part of the program. It not only trains the muscles, but it also engages the nervous system to create explosive movements, which is required for effectiveness on the court.

Basketball Workout

Modality	Exercise	Page
Dynamic warm-up	Relaxed skip series	75
Dynamic warm-up	Both-arms-up skip	76
Dynamic warm-up	Opposite-arm, opposite-leg skip	77
Dynamic warm-up	Wide skip	78
Joint articulation series	Ankles series	66
Joint articulation series	Knee circle	68
Joint articulation series	Hip flexion and extension	69
Olympic lifts	High pull	207
Olympic lifts	Snatch	211
Dumbbell	Dumbbell squat	196
Dumbbell	Dumbbell overhead press	201
Pilates	Standing roll-down	147
Pilates	Leg pull	136
Pilates	Single-leg kick	132
Pilates	Double-leg kick	133
Pilates	Roll-up	118
Pilates	Mermaid	138
Medicine ball	Crunch	170
Medicine ball	Diagonal	169
Medicine ball	Side tap	171
Medicine ball	Prone series	172

Impact Sports
(Football, Rugby, Boxing and Mixed Martial Arts)

Impact sports definitely do a number on your entire body. To challenge your allover fitness, focus on the following exercises for injury prevention.

Football

The game is all about giving and receiving impact. This program will prepare you for that.

Football Workout

Exercise	Modality	Page
Foam roller	Shoulder roll	42
Foam roller	Chest opener	43
Foam roller	Quadriceps release	53
Foam roller	IT band release	52
Foam roller	Hamstring stretch	50
Dynamic warm-up	Relaxed skip series	75
Dynamic warm-up	Jumping jack skip	77
Dynamic warm-up	Wide skip	78
Dynamic warm-up	Lateral skip	80
Olympic lifts	Hang clean	209
Dumbbell	Dumbbell squat	196
Dumbbell	Dumbbell RDL	198
Olympic lifts	Jerk and push press	213
Pilates	Hundreds	111
Pilates	Hamstring pull	116
Pilates	Roll-up	118
Pilates	Spine twist	120
Pilates	Side kick series: • Lift and lower • Front and back kick • Circle	123

Rugby

Very much like football, rugby is an impact sport and needs to be trained that way. We have included the snatch in this workout; you can easily put a clean component behind it as well.

Rugby Workout

Exercise	Modality	Page
Foam roller	Nervous system activation	40
Foam roller	Quadriceps release	53
Foam roller	IT band release	52
Foam roller	Calf stretch	51
Dynamic warm-up	Relaxed skip series	75
Dynamic warm-up	Jumping jack skip	77
Dynamic warm-up	Wide skip	78
Dynamic warm-up	Lateral skip	80
Pilates	Hundreds	111
Pilates	Double-leg stretch	114
Pilates	Hamstring pull	116
Pilates	Mermaid	138
Pilates	Spine twist	120
Pilates	Double-leg kick	133
Pilates	Neck pull	119
Pilates	Saw	122
Pilates	Side-kick series: • Lift and lower • Front and back kick • Side-lying clam	123
Olympic lifts	Snatch	211
Dumbbell	Dumbbell RDL	198
Dumbbell	Dumbbell squat	196
Dumbbell	Dumbbell row	199

Boxing and Mixed Martial Arts

Strength and power are the components behind this program. It's very effective.

Boxing and Mixed Martial Arts Workout

Exercise	Modality	Page
Joint articulation series	Ankles series	66
Joint articulation series	Knee circle	68
Joint articulation series	Hip flexion and extension	69
Joint articulation series	Chin extension and flexion	71
Pilates	Hundreds	111
Pilates	Single-leg stretch	113
Pilates	Double-leg stretch	114
Pilates	Teaser	144
Pilates	Leg pull front	142
Pilates	Swimming	131
Pilates	Standing roll-down	147
Medicine ball	Squat	162
Medicine ball	Reverse lunge	163
Medicine ball	Forward lunge	164
Olympic lifts	Hang clean	209
Dumbbell	Dumbbell squat	196
Dumbbell	Dumbbell RDL	198
Dumbbell	Dumbbell overhead press	201

As we said in the beginning of the book, this is your go-to manual for program and exercise ideas. By using the material in each chapter, coaches and athletes will be able to create thousands of programs. The programs we outlined are just a sampling of what is possible. Remember, not every exercise is appropriate for every athlete. Each program that you are creating for the day no matter how long or short the workout will be should include the following: activating the nervous system, warming up the body, the work phase, core, and stretch. All Beyond Motion athletes no matter age or sport follow this pattern. And the single most important piece of information we can give you is that it is imperative to create a strong, stable, flexible base to become a successful mover and that takes time. The key to developing a strong foundation is to advance your athlete only when they are ready and to build in adequate recovery; this will minimize injury.

Al Vermeil once told me "You can't coach what you haven't felt." In other words, if you're going to coach an athlete through the movements in this book, make sure you have experienced and perfected them first. For instance, the feeling of meeting the bar in a good hang clean is incredible.

Make sure your coaching is on par with your experience.

GLOSSARY

abdominals or abs—The muscles in the front of or in the abdomen. Your rectus abdominals (rectus abdominis, commonly referred to as a six-pack), obliques, and transverse abdominals create your abdominal area. In Pilates this is referred to as part of your powerhouse.

anterior pelvic tilt—In this position, the front of the pelvis drops and the back of the pelvis rises. This happens when the hip flexors shorten and the hip extensors lengthen. (Stand tall and place your hands at your pelvic girdle. Think of the Liberty Bell as you tip your pelvis back, allowing the lumbar portion of your spine to arch.)

anterior superior iliac spine (ASIS)—The bony prominence at the top and front of the pelvis. People often refer to it incorrectly as the hip bone. It is easy to find when you are lying on your back because the bone tends to stick out when you are in this position.

axial elongation—Your posture and the length of your spine. Think of this as the longest line from the crown of your head to your tailbone. Allow the natural curves in your spine, but without feeling swaybacked and with no section of your spine feeling compressed.

cervical spine—The cervical spine, or neck, begins at the base of the skull and is made up of seven vertebrae. The lower segment connects to the thoracic area of your spine. The first cervical vertebra is called the atlas and rotates around part of the second vertebra, your axis. This is the area responsible for the rotation of your neck and head. The seven vertebrae of the cervical spine are connected in the back by paired facet joints, which allow for forward and backward extension as well as twisting movements. These facet joints can wear down over time and lead to cervical spinal stenosis or osteoarthritis.

iliotibial (IT) band—The IT band stabilizes the knee and assists in abduction. It begins at the side of the iliac crest and attaches to a small muscle called the tensor fasciae latae (TFL). It runs along the lateral side of the thigh and across the knee joint, where it attaches to the tibia.

lumbar spine—The five vertebrae of the lumbar spine (L1–L5) are the biggest unfused vertebrae in the spinal column, enabling them to support the weight of the entire torso. At the same time, the lumbar spine is highly flexible, providing for mobility in many different planes, including flexion, extension, side bending, and rotation.

neutral pelvis—The most natural alignment of the pelvis. You should not feel tucked under, arched back, or tilted to one side. In this position, your pelvis should be level. Trace a triangle from one side of your iliac crest across your belly button to the other side, down to your pubic bone and up to the other side of your iliac crest. The triangle should be level, and not tipped at any point.

neutral spine—A balanced spine that maintains its natural curves. Pilates encourages a person to identify and achieve a neutral spine. A misaligned spine causes compensation in muscles, creating undue stress, fatigue, pain, inefficient movement, and potential injury.

obliques—The internal and external oblique muscles run along the side and front of the abdomen. The external oblique muscle is one of the outermost abdominal muscles, extending from the lower half of the ribs around and down to the pelvis. The obliques allow your body to rotate and bend to the side.

pelvic floor—The pelvic floor is the muscular structure that lines the bottom of the pelvis. The pelvic floor is part of the core and contributes to postural alignment and stability and relates synergistically to the diaphragm. It helps to distribute the weight and pressure of the internal organs and relates to the musculature of the hips and deep transverse abdominals (TA).

piriformis—A small muscle located deep in the glutes, behind the gluteus maximus. It runs diagonally from the lower spine to the upper surface of the femur. The sciatic nerve runs under or through the muscle. The piriformis helps your hip rotate and assists in rotating the leg and foot outward.

posterior pelvic tilt—In this position the front of the pelvis rises and the back of the pelvis drops. This happens when the hip flexors lengthen and the hip extensors shorten. Think of the Liberty Bell as you allow your pelvis to tip so that the tailbone tucks under you and your hips shift forward.

posterior superior iliac spine (PSIS)—This part of the sacral triangle ranges from the outer tip of one side of the iliac crest, across the sacroiliac (SI) joint to the other side, and tracing down to the coccyx. The posterior superior iliac spine serves as the attachment of the oblique portion of the posterior sacroiliac ligaments and the multifidus.

prone—Lying facedown or facing downward as in a quadruped position.

rectus abdominals (or rectus abdominis)—Also known as abs or six-pack. This paired muscle runs vertically on each side of the anterior wall of the abdomen, and the right and left side are separated at the midline by a band of connective tissue called the linea alba.

sacroiliac (SI) joint—The joint in the bony pelvis between the sacrum and the ilium of the pelvis. The bones are joined by strong ligaments. The sacrum supports the spine and is supported in turn by an ilium on each side. There is an SI joint on each side of the body.

sacrum—This is the triangular bone at the base of the spine between the ilia of the posterior pelvis. The top of the sacrum is referred to as the sacral base. The bottom is referred to as the apex, tailbone, or coccyx, which reinforces the posterior pelvic floor. The sacrum consists of five fused bones and is the portion of the spine that does not rotate.

supine—Lying faceup.

thoracic spine—Twelve vertebrae (T1–T12) make up the thoracic portion of the spine, which runs from the top of the shoulder girdle to the lowest rib. These vertebrae are firmly attached to the ribs and sternum (breastbone) and allow the body to twist and bend.

transverse abdominals (TA)—These muscles form the deepest layer of the abdominals and are most efficiently activated by drawing the navel back toward the spine. The job of the transverse abdominals is to increase intraabdominal pressure and control the mobility of the lumbar spine.

ABOUT THE AUTHORS

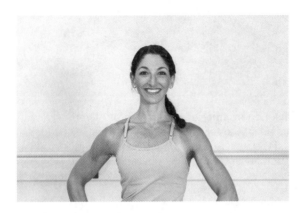

Amy Lademann, PMA®-CPT, and her husband Rick are the Founders of BEYOND MOTION®, a state of the art performance facility with their headquarters in Naples, Florida. BEYOND MOTION® is designed to combine the worlds of athlete performance and Pilates. Since 2009, they have been recognized as leaders in the industry training elite and professional athletes alike.

Amy danced as a child and at sixteen, she began her fitness career by becoming certified in aerobics and step aerobics. Her passion for fitness fueled her quest for knowledge, so throughout the next two decades she earned additional certifications in the Nia Technique, Bellatone, Barre, Zumba (and other dance fitness programs), as well as Yoga. Unfortunately, during her twenties Amy developed severe sciatica and back issues. After trying everything to alleviate her discomfort, she discovered Pilates. She was instantly hooked. Pilates was the one thing that finally helped heal her pain. She began her Pilates career with Polestar in 2001 and continued her education through a variety of contemporary Pilates methods, including her certifications in the MOTR and Bodhi through Balanced Body. In 2016 Amy partnered with the esteemed Pilates Education Institute to create BEYOND MOTION's comprehensive Pilates Teacher Training Program and has been nicknamed the "teacher's teacher" by her students.

Looking to raise her own bar, in 2017 Amy competed in her first figure and bikini competitions through the NGA (National Gym Association), a drug-free bodybuilding organization. At her first competition, she won first place in Figure Debut for the first time on stage, Figure Masters for the over 35-year-old category, Figure Open for every age and level, and second place in Bikini Open. She also earned her Pro Card, which meant she could compete at the pro level in figure competitions. In 2018, she competed again on an even larger stage and earned second and third place in her divisions. Striving to improve one's best self is just as important to her now as it was all those years ago.

Pilates and Conditioning for Athletes: An Integrated Approach to Performance and Recovery, will be Amy and Rick's first book. To learn more about Amy and BEYOND MOTION® visit www.go2beyondmotion.com.

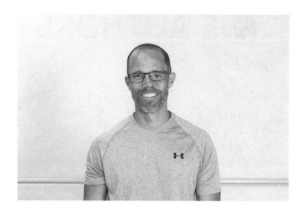

While in his 20s, **Rick Lademann** began working for Al Vermeil and the World Champion Chicago Bulls, where he stayed for three years. After that, he headed to Colorado Springs, where he worked at the United States Olympic Training Center for USA Weightlifting under the care of former Romanian Olympic weightlifter Dragomir Cioroslan. Rick lived on the campus for two years and was instrumental in developing the junior squad and programming volume numbers for our Olympic Athletes.

He then expanded his career even further when he went to the U.S. Air Force Academy, also in Colorado, to assist the football team with their speed and strength program. During this time, he also worked with the USA Figure Skating team at the Colorado Springs World Arena. Rick's teaching of core awareness and how to provide power became essential for many of the Olympic Competitors.

After that, Rick worked with internationally recognized orthopedic surgeons at the Steadman Hawkins Clinic as the strength and conditioning consultant. It was at the clinic where Rick handled post physical therapy on all their professional athletes, specifically the Colorado Rockies. This opportunity led to Rick becoming the primary performance coach for baseball player Larry Walker, the only Rockies player ever to win the National League MVP award. Even famed sportswriter Ken Rosenthal noticed a change in Walker's performance after Rick began his work, stating that the program Rick created made such a difference in Walker's performance that it was evident from the start of spring training.

Rick then served as the strength coach at the University of California, Berkley, where he was instrumental in helping the Cal rugby team win a national championship in 2003. In addition to rugby, Rick served the men's and women's tennis, baseball, and basketball teams.

Since the early 2000s, Rick has become the primary strength and speed coach for over 100 MLB, NBA, NFL, tennis, and golf athletes. Known for his in-depth knowledge of the body, he is considered a unique resource in the field and is sought out by many athletes during their off-season.

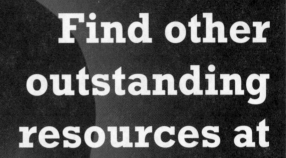

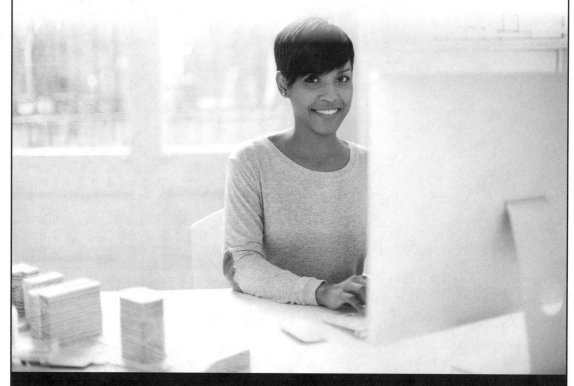
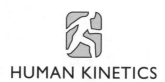